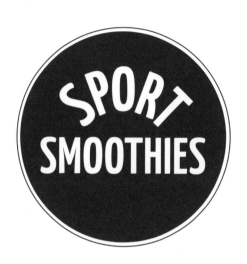

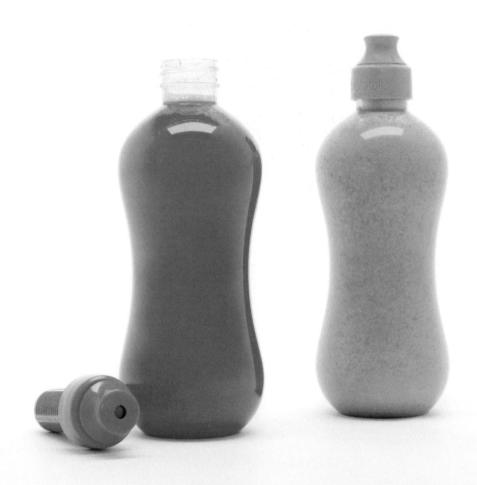

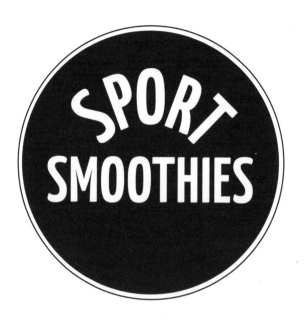

MORE THAN
65 RECIPES
TO BOOST YOUR
WORKOUTS & RECOVERY

Fern Green

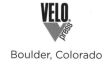

Boulder, Colorado

CONTENTS

6 *Introduction*
9 *Fueling Your Body for Sport*

Pre-Workout

14 Coconut Date
16 Blue Apple
18 Papaya Pine
20 Choc Espresso
22 Açai Seng
24 Coco Berry
26 Figgy Water
28 Piña Coco Lada
30 Yo Strawberries
32 Berry Scoop
34 Blue Egg
36 Pear Pro
38 Green Up
40 Banana Oat
42 Match Fit Maca
44 Beet Out
46 Chia Tea
48 Peanut Spice

Post-Workout & Recovery

52 Pom Flax-tastic
54 Brocco Bana
56 Chia Charge
58 Orangavo
60 Cherry Bomb
62 Grape Trifecta
64 Nut Better
66 Pink Basil
68 Green Peach
70 Mango-Yo
72 Kale Kiwi Tea
74 Sweet-Kea
76 Almond Joy
78 Raspberry Date
80 Cacao Delight
82 Tropical Turmeric
84 Green Monster
86 Pollen Berry

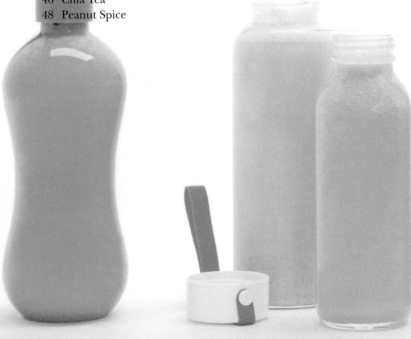

Muscle-Building

90 Oat & Tofu
92 Coco Melon
94 Magic Mango
96 Fruity Kale
98 Papaya Passion
100 Kiwi Raspberry
102 Oaty Apple
104 Caribbean Kick
106 Green Protein
108 Loca Mocha
110 Cranberry Pro
112 Blue Cashew
114 Pumpkin Patch
116 Banana Nut
118 Super Goji
120 Piña Spirulina
122 Peanut Chia

Carb-Loading

126 Peach Carbler
128 Cacao Flax
130 Sweet Potato Jive
132 Spinachia
134 Almond Load
136 Branberry Rocket
138 Back in Black
140 Nutty Boom
142 Orange Tornado
144 Peachellini
146 Oat Me Up
148 Sweet Papaya Poyo
150 Veggie Beet
152 Sweet Potana
154 Buckwheat Bang
156 Orangey Apricot

158 *Index*

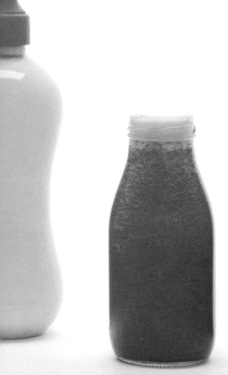

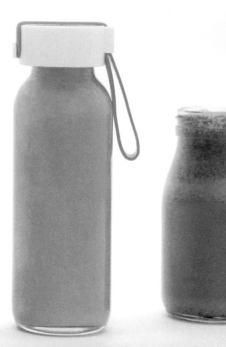

INTRODUCTION

Whether you compete in sports such as cycling, running, swimming, or working out at the gym, it all requires energy. The foods that you eat on a daily basis are your body's primary source of energy, so getting the right balance of nutrients is essential to fueling your exercise.

The foods you eat must fuel both your body and mind, keeping your muscles energized and your brain focused and alert. This means digesting quality, healthy calories to achieve an optimal mix of macronutrients— carbohydrates, fats, and protein. However, finding the time to prepare and eat healthily can be difficult. The smoothies in this book take into account all of an athlete's needs, including pre- and post-workout, muscle-building and carb-loading, serving up the essential ingredients at the right time to complement your workout and fuel your body.

Smoothies provide a fast and efficient way to boost your daily intake of healthy calories and give your brain and body the fuel needed for optimal performance. Pre-workout and carb-loading smoothies supply your body with essential hydration and the quality calories required to fuel the body for exercise or a big event without overloading the stomach. Post-workout, recovery, and muscle-building smoothies work to top off glycogen stores after every effort, whether in day-to-day training or following a particularly intense effort. With more than 65 no-fuss recipes to choose from, *Sport Smoothies* will fuel your workouts, promote muscle repair, and aid recovery, giving you an easy and delicious alternative to the bulky meals that so often lead to discomfort.

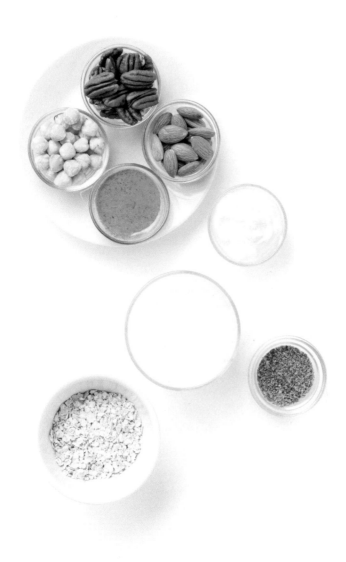

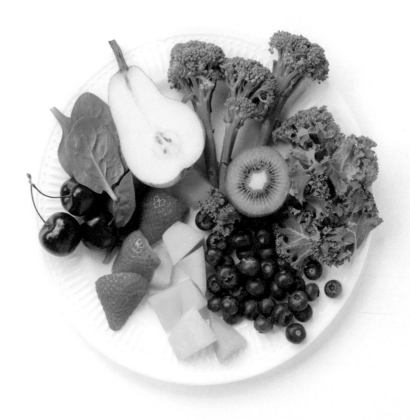

FUELING YOUR BODY FOR SPORT

Carbohydrates, fats, and protein all work to fuel your body. When you know the role each macronutrient plays, you can make better decisions about what foods to eat and when to eat them. You'll find the smoothies grouped accordingly, and at the start of each section you can review the nutritional information for each one. This information can be useful in meeting the demands of everyday training, and particularly in preparation for competition or racing.

Carbohydrates

This macronutrient is the body's primary source of energy and is made up of two types: simple carbohydrates and complex carbohydrates. Simple carbohydrates include sugary foods, fruit, milk products, select refined grains, and simple sugars. Complex carbohydrates include many vegetables and starchy foods such as whole grain breads, potatoes, cereals, pastas, and rice.

All carbohydrates must be converted to glucose and glycogen before they can be used as fuel for your body. Complex carbohydrates are broken down more slowly than simple carbohydrates, so they provide a slower release of energy. Whether you are swimming, cycling, or running, your working muscles are fueled by glucose in the blood and by glycogen stores in the liver and muscles. When your body has a sufficient supply of glucose, carbohydrates are converted to glycogen and stored. When glucose is in short supply, glycogen is converted to glucose and made ready for use. Post-workout, it is a good idea to replenish your glycogen stores, which will boost your energy levels for the rest of the day.

FOODS HIGH IN CARBOHYDRATES

 Fruits. Most fruits provide a quick and healthy source of energy, making them good fuel for endurance sports. Strawberries, pears, mangoes, bananas, kiwi, cherries, apricots, and blueberries are just some of the fruits high in carbohydrates.

 Dark Green Leafy Vegetables. Kale, broccoli, and spinach are nutritionally dense and are ideal in green smoothies. The added fiber helps to slow the absorption of sugar to provide the body with a slow, steady release of energy, which leads to improved physical and mental alertness.

 Rice & Oats. Rice milk and oats also top off glycogen stores with the slow-release energy that fuels your body for sport.

Fats

There are two types of fat: saturated and unsaturated. Saturated fats are the unhealthy fats found in foods such as butter, cheese, and fatty meats, while unsaturated fats are the healthier fats found in vegetable oils, fish oils, nuts, seeds, and avocados.

We all need fat in our diet. Not all fats are equal, but like carbohydrates, fats can provide the body with energy. In fact, fats yield 9 calories per gram compared to only 4 calories per gram of carbohydrates. However, fat is a much slower source of energy so when you are exercising hard, your body turns to glycogen stores for a more immediate release of energy. During longer duration, steady-paced efforts, your body tries to conserve as much of its glycogen reserves as possible, instead accessing fat stores for energy.

Your body will convert excess carbohydrate and protein in your diet into fat, but it cannot manufacture certain essential unsaturated fats—the foods you eat are your body's only supply of these healthy fats. The essential fatty acids are omega-3, found in fish, flax seeds, and walnuts, and omega-6, found in vegetable oils, such as olive oil and sunflower oil. Fats act as a carrier for fat-soluble vitamins, including vitamins A, D, K, and E, and they provide insulation and protection for your body.

Flaxseeds. High in omega-3 fatty acids, flaxseeds also contain B vitamins, magnesium, and manganese. B vitamins are involved in the release of energy from food; magnesium plays an important role in muscles contraction; and manganese is a vital component of many enzymes involved in energy production.

Peanut Butter. Peanuts are high in healthy unsaturated fats and calorically dense. They also contain B vitamins, phosphorus, iron, copper, potassium, and vitamin E. Copper helps to protect against free radical damage and plays an important role in helping the body to absorb iron from food.

Almond Butter. Almonds are a good source of vitamin E and antioxidants, which give the immune system a boost. They also contribute to a healthy heart.

Protein

Protein is essential for muscle building. It can be used as a source of energy, but this would only be the case if your body's glycogen stores were totally depleted. Protein is also essential for healthy tissue growth and repair, which is necessary as regular exercise can cause repetitive wear and tear of soft tissue.

FOODS HIGH IN PROTEIN

Plant Milk. Unsweetened, fortified milk alternatives can be a great source of high-quality protein, calcium, zinc, and phosphorus. There is a wide variety of plant milks available, and they can be used interchangeably in smoothies.

Yogurt. A good source of calcium and phosphorus to help strengthen bones, yogurt adds a rich and creamy texture to a smoothie. Choose plain dairy or dairy-free yogurts.

Oats. Not only are oats a source of complex carbohydrates, they also contain fiber and are relatively high in protein, making them a great addition to a smoothie.

PRE-WORKOUT

These smoothies are packed full of nutrient-dense ingredients to keep you fueled up for any type of exercise. Whether you are heading out for a run, a spin class, or a training session at the gym, these pre-workout smoothies will supply the energy you need.

PRE-WORKOUT SMOOTHIES	CALORIES	PROTEIN (G)	FAT (G)	CARBS (G)	FIBER (G)	SODIUM (MG)
Coconut Date (p. 14)	512	4	2	132	13	100
Blue Apple (p. 16)	343	2	1	87	7	12
Papaya Pine (p. 18)	363	4	4	85	8	13
Choc Espresso (p. 20)	364	2	4	73	6	32
Açai Seng (p. 22)	230	1	1	62	6	43
Coco Berry (p. 24)	541	8	9	116	15	53
Figgy Water (p. 26)	493	4	1	154	13	26
Piña Coco Lada (p. 28)	382	16	1	81	12	7
Yo Strawberries (p. 30)	388	4	11	78	11	50
Berry Scoop (p. 32)	232	22	3	32	7	1
Blue Egg (p. 34)	426	11	31	30	11	234
Pear Pro (p. 36)	404	4	6	94	21	105
Green Up (p. 38)	152	5	<1	34	4	102
Banana Oat (p. 40)	605	15	15	110	16	162
Match Fit Maca (p. 42)	226	5	3	50	7	183
Beet Out (p. 44)	130	2	<1	29	3	124
Chia Tea (p. 46)	136	2	4	23	5	<5
Peanut Spice (p. 48)	439	10	13	62	9	223

COCONUT DATE

Serves: 1 | Preparation: 5 minutes

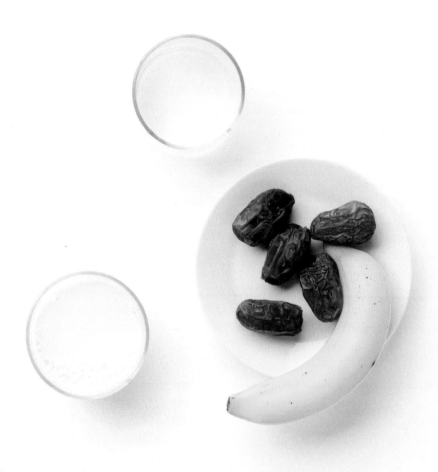

YOU NEED

1 cup coconut water • ½ cup almond milk
5 Medjool dates, pitted • 1 banana, peeled and chopped

Dates are high in fiber, which can help lower cholesterol.

E *Energy boosting*   **M** *Mineral enriching*   **V** *Vitamin boosting*

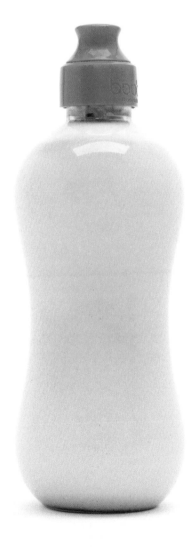

Place all the ingredients in a blender and blend until smooth.

BLUE APPLE

Serves: 1 | Preparation: 5 minutes

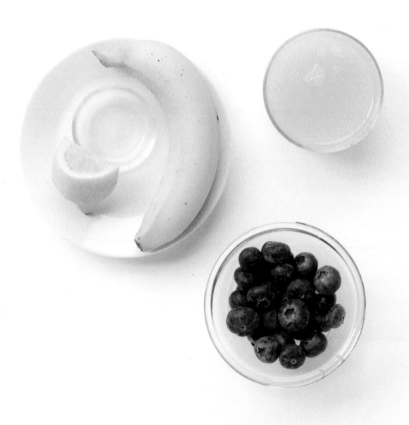

YOU NEED

1 cup fresh apple juice • 1 cup blueberries • 1 banana, peeled and chopped
¼ cup coconut water • juice of ¼ lemon

Apples contain enzymes that help break down carbohydrates and regulate blood sugar levels.

V *Vitamin boosting*   **H** *Hydrating*   **S** *Skin enhancing*

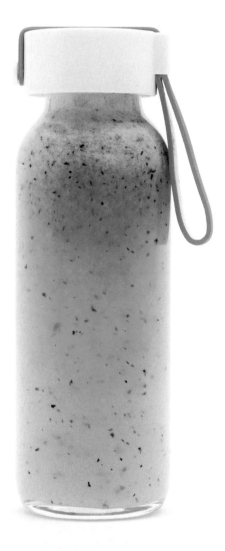

Place all the ingredients in a blender and blend until smooth.

PAPAYA PINE

Serves: 1 | Preparation: 5 minutes

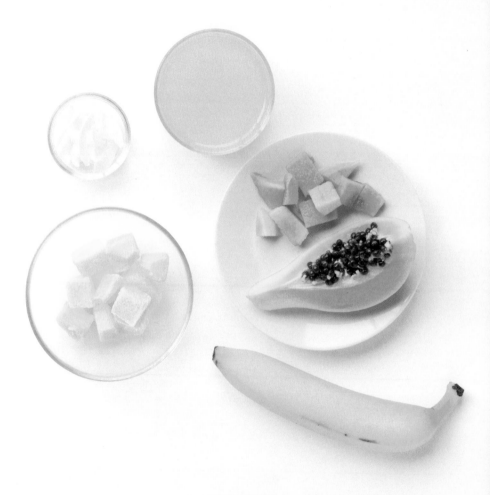

YOU NEED

1 cup pineapple juice • 1 banana, peeled and chopped
½ cup papaya, peeled, seeded, and chopped
½ mango, peeled and chopped • 1 tablespoon dried coconut flakes

Pineapple is high in vitamin C, which is vital for the immune system.

D *Aids digestion* **V** *Vitamin boosting* **M** *Mineral enriching*

Place all the ingredients in a blender and blend until smooth.

CHOC ESPRESSO

Serves: 1 | Preparation: 5 minutes

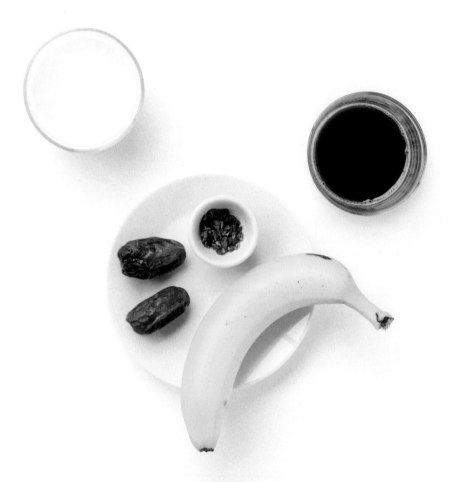

YOU NEED

1 cup cashew milk • 1 shot (1 oz.) espresso coffee, chilled
1 banana, peeled and chopped • ½ tablespoon cacao nibs
2 Medjool dates, pitted

Cashew milk contains vitamin K, which is essential for helping blood clot and building strong bones.

B *Blood stimulating* **E** *Energy boosting* **P** *Protein boosting*

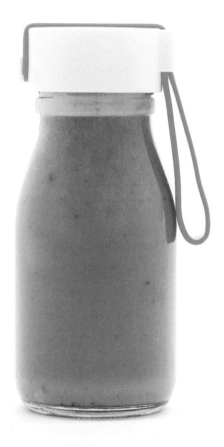

Place all the ingredients in a blender and blend until smooth.

AÇAI SENG

Serves: 1 | Preparation: 5 minutes

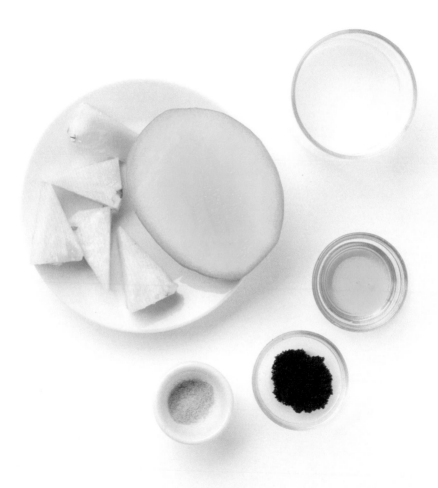

YOU NEED

½ cup mango, peeled and cut into chunks • ½ cup pineapple chunks
1 cup coconut water • 1 tablespoon açai powder • 1 tablespoon raw honey
½ teaspoon ginseng powder

Açai berries contain plant sterols, compounds that interfere with the body's ability to absorb cholesterol from food, thereby reducing overall levels.

(V) *Vitamin boosting*   **(E)** *Energy boosting*   **(H)** *Hydrating*

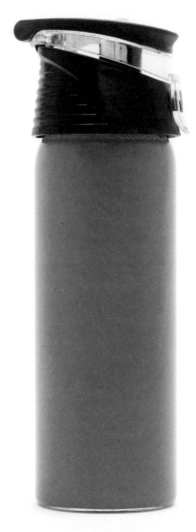

Place all the ingredients in a blender with ⅓ cup water
and blend until smooth.

COCO BERRY

Serves: 1 | Preparation: 5 minutes

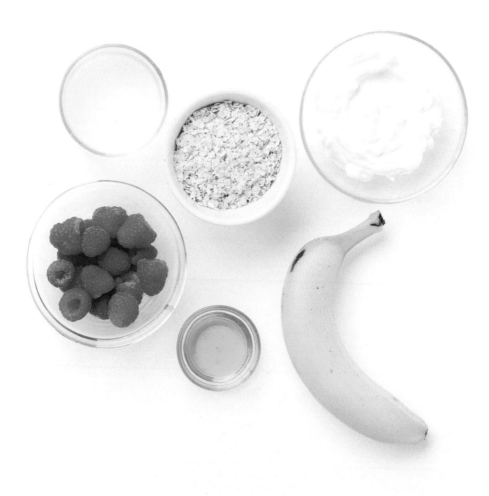

YOU NEED

1 cup coconut water • ½ cup raspberries • 1 banana, peeled and chopped
½ cup rolled oats • ¼ cup coconut yogurt • 1 tablespoon raw honey

Rolled oats contain a unique type of fiber, beta glucan, which can aid heart health.

Ⓥ Vitamin boosting *Ⓗ Hydrating* *Ⓜ Mineral enriching*

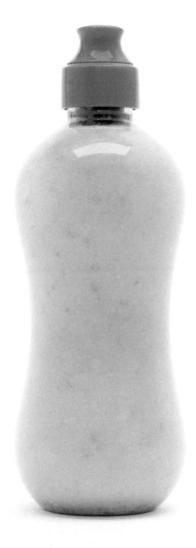

Place all the ingredients in a blender and blend until smooth.

FIGGY WATER

Serves: 1 | Preparation: 5 minutes

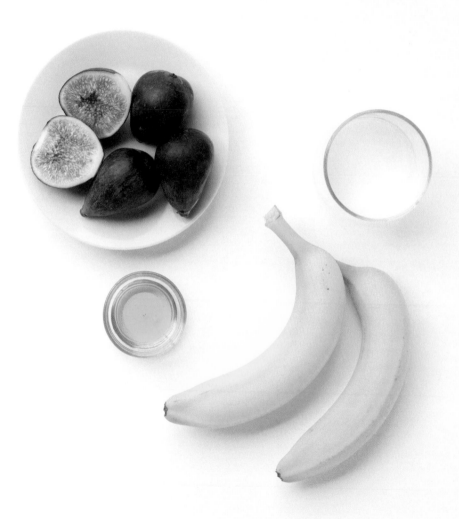

YOU NEED

1 cup coconut water • 2 bananas, peeled and chopped
4 figs, halved • 1 tablespoon agave nectar

Figs promote bone density as they contain a high amount of calcium.

D *Aids digestion*   **H** *Hydrating*   **M** *Mineral enriching*

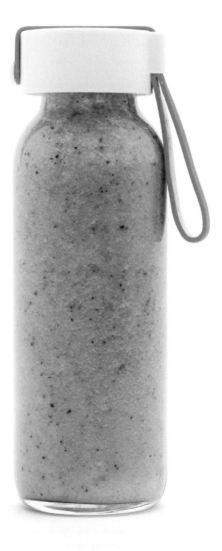

Place all the ingredients in a blender and blend until smooth.

PIÑA COCO LADA

Serves: 1 | Preparation: 5 minutes

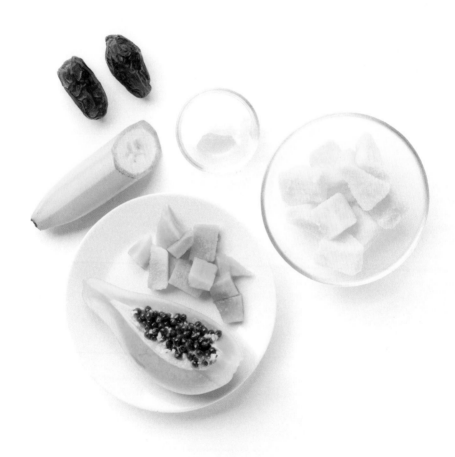

YOU NEED

1 cup pineapple chunks • ½ banana, peeled and chopped
½ cup papaya, peeled, seeded, and cut into chunks
2 Medjool dates, pitted • 1 tablespoon coconut oil

Pineapple contains the enzyme bromelain, which can help to reduce inflammation in joints and muscles.

Ⓥ *Vitamin boosting*   Ⓜ *Mineral enriching*   Ⓓ *Aids digestion*

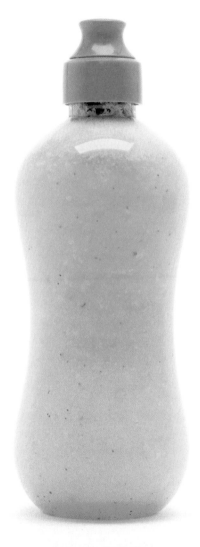

Place all the ingredients in a blender with ⅓ cup water and blend until smooth.

YO STRAWBERRIES

Serves: 1 | Preparation: 5 minutes

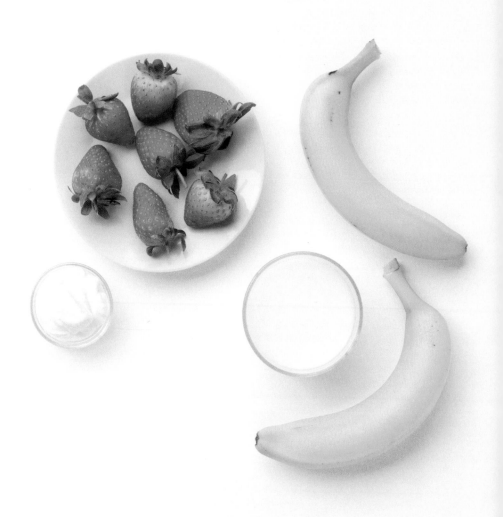

YOU NEED

1 cup coconut milk • ½ cup strawberries, hulled
2 bananas, peeled and chopped • ¼ cup coconut yogurt

Strawberries are an excellent source of vitamins C and K and provide a good dose of fiber, folic acid, manganese, and potassium.

B *Bone strengthening*   **V** *Vitamin boosting*   **I** *Immunity boosting*

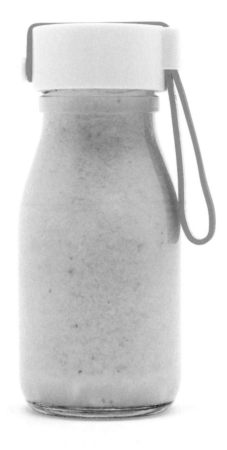

Place all the ingredients in a blender and blend until smooth.

BERRY SCOOP

Serves: 1 | Preparation: 5 minutes

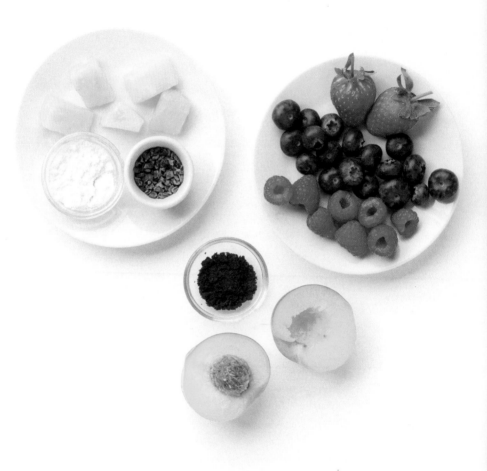

YOU NEED

¾ cup mixed berries • 1 peach, pitted and chopped
¼ cup pineapple chunks • 1 scoop protein powder
½ tablespoon cacao nibs • 1 teaspoon açai powder

Berries are a great source of fiber, which helps aid digestion.

V *Vitamin boosting* **B** *Blood stimulating* **I** *Immunity boosting*

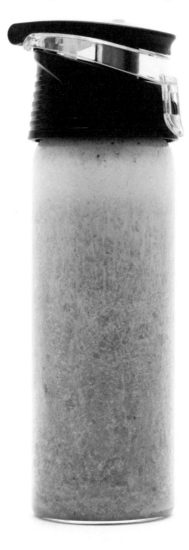

Place all the ingredients in a blender with 1 cup water and blend until smooth.

BLUE EGG

Serves: 1 | Preparation: 5 minutes

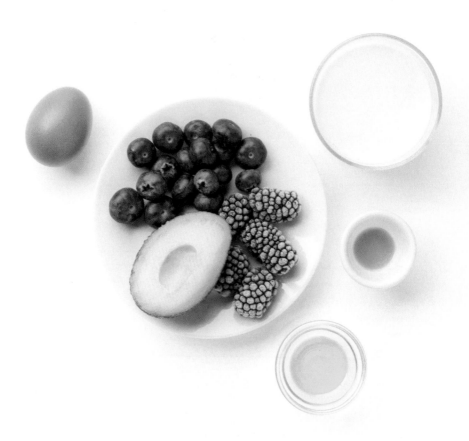

YOU NEED

1 cup almond milk • ⅔ cup blueberries • ⅓ cup blackberries (fresh or frozen)
1 raw organic egg • ½ small avocado, pitted and peeled
1 tablespoon flaxseed oil • ¼ teaspoon pure vanilla extract

Blueberries are packed with antioxidants called anthocyanins, which may help keep your memory sharp as you age.

P *Protein boosting* **S** *Skin enhancing* **B** *Bone strengthening*

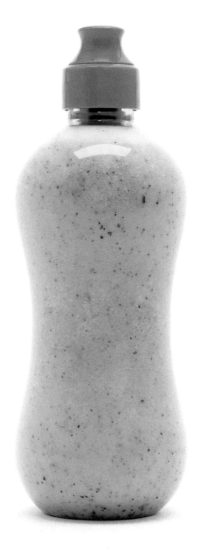

Place all the ingredients in a blender and blend until smooth.

PEAR PRO

Serves: 1 | Preparation: 5 minutes

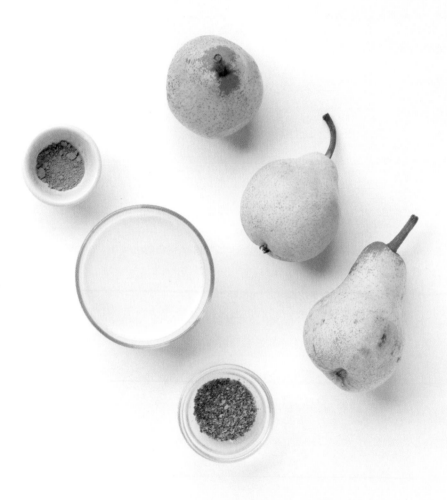

YOU NEED

1 cup almond milk • 3 pears, peeled, cored, and chopped
½ teaspoon matcha (green tea) powder • 1 tablespoon ground flaxseed

Pears are a good source of minerals, such as copper, iron, potassium, manganese, and magnesium, as well as B-complex vitamins including folates and riboflavin.

(V) *Vitamin boosting*   **(M)** *Mineral enriching*   **(A)** *Anti-inflammatory*

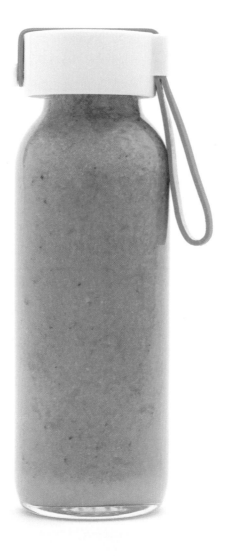

Place all the ingredients in a blender and blend until smooth.

GREEN UP

Serves: 1 | Preparation: 5 minutes

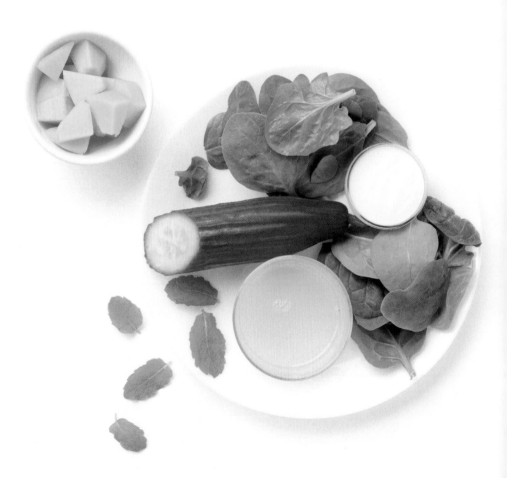

YOU NEED

1 cup cantaloupe, cut into chunks • 5 mint leaves
2 handfuls of baby spinach • ½ cucumber, cut into chunks
¼ cup fresh apple juice • 2 tablespoons plain yogurt

Cantaloupe is a great source of potassium and B vitamins.

H *Hydrating* **V** *Vitamin boosting* **B** *Brain boosting*

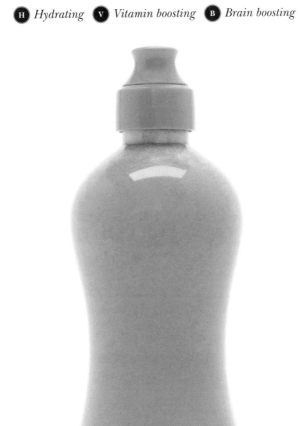

Place all the ingredients in a blender with 1 cup water and blend until smooth.

BANANA OAT

Serves: 1 | Preparation: 5 minutes

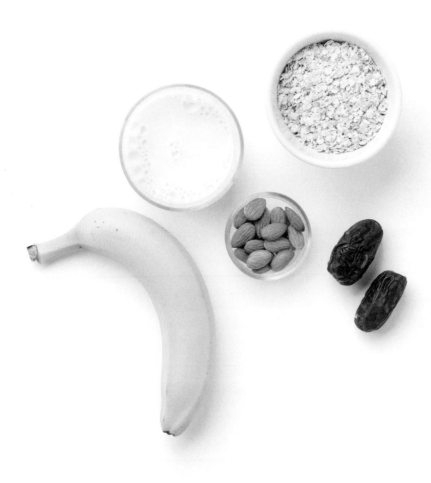

YOU NEED

1 cup almond milk • ⅔ cup rolled oats • 1 banana, peeled and chopped
2 Medjool dates, pitted • 1 tablespoon raw almonds

Bananas are a great source of potassium, which is an essential mineral for maintaining proper heart function and regulating blood pressure.

(P) *Protein boosting*　**(S)** *Skin enhancing*　**(M)** *Mineral enriching*

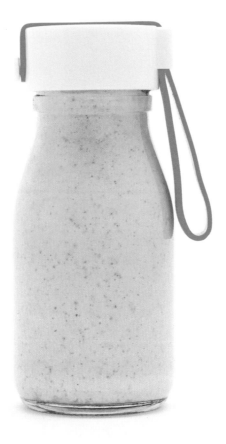

Place all the ingredients in a blender and blend until smooth.

MATCH FIT MACA

Serves: 1 | *Preparation: 5 minutes*

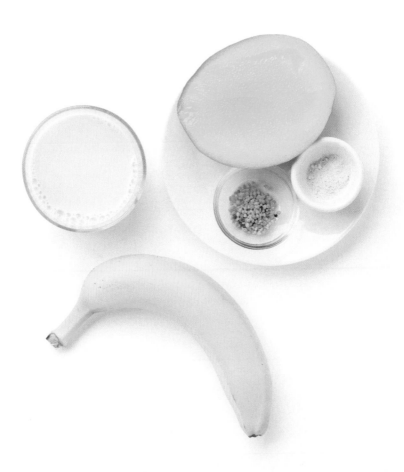

YOU NEED

1 cup almond milk • 1 banana, peeled and chopped
½ mango, peeled and chopped • 1 teaspoon maca powder
1 teaspoon bee pollen

Maca is rich in vitamins B, C, and E.

V *Vitamin boosting* **B** *Bone strengthening* **E** *Energy boosting*

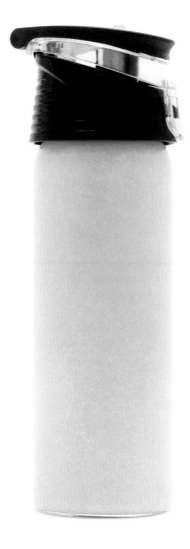

Place all the ingredients in a blender and blend until smooth.

BEET OUT

Serves: 1 | Preparation: 5 minutes

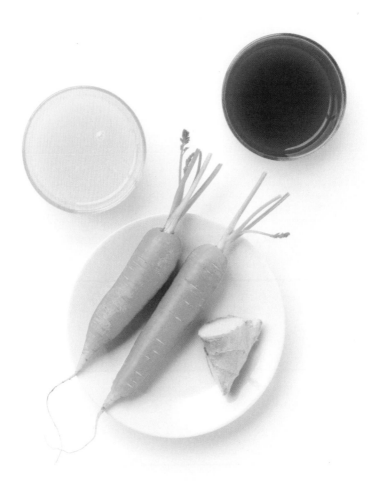

YOU NEED

⅓ cup beet juice • 2 carrots, peeled and chopped
1-inch piece of ginger, peeled • ⅓ cup fresh apple juice

Beets are a good source of iron and folate, and there is research suggesting beet juice can boost exercise performance and even heart health.

M *Mineral enriching*   **V** *Vitamin boosting*   **B** *Blood stimulating*

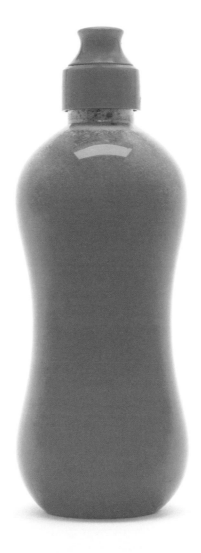

Place all the ingredients in a blender with ½ cup water and blend until smooth.

CHIA TEA

Serves: 2–3 | Preparation: 15 minutes

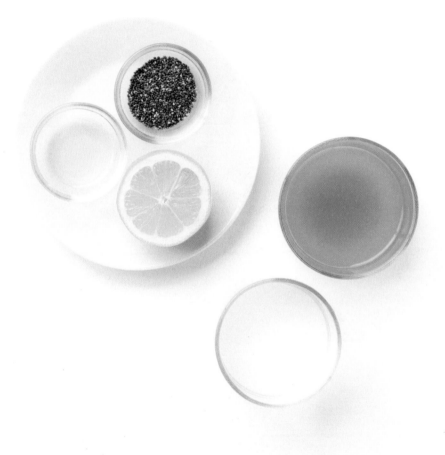

YOU NEED

1 cup green tea, chilled • 1 cup coconut water
juice of 1 lemon • 1 tablespoon chia seeds

Chia seeds are rich in polyunsaturated fats, especially omega-3 fatty acids.

A *Anti-inflammatory* **V** *Vitamin boosting* **H** *Hydrating*

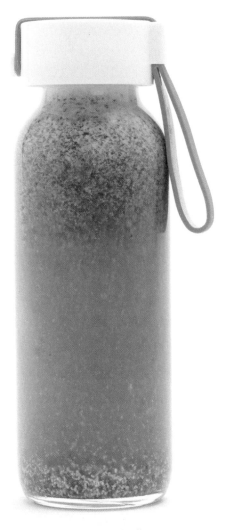

Pour all the ingredients into a jug with 1 cup water and leave to stand for 10 minutes. This encourages the chia seeds to become gelatinous.

PEANUT SPICE

Serves: 1 | Preparation: 5 minutes

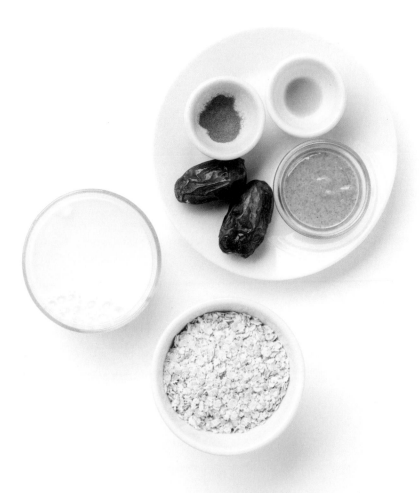

YOU NEED

1 cup almond milk • ⅓ cup rolled oats
1 tablespoon smooth natural peanut butter • 2 Medjool dates, pitted
a pinch of ground cinnamon • ½ teaspoon pure vanilla extract

Peanut butter contains satiating fat and is an excellent source of magnesium, a critical nutrient for healthy muscle function.

P *Protein boosting*   **D** *Aids digestion*   **B** *Bone strengthening*

Place all the ingredients in a blender and blend until smooth.

POST-WORKOUT & RECOVERY

After a long training session or a race,
it helps to take in protein and carbs—
replacing all that good stuff you just used up.
After less strenuous efforts, reach for
a lighter smoothie with the nutrients to
promote holistic recovery and wellness.
Done right, recovery defends against soreness,
stiffness, and general fatigue.

POST-WORKOUT & RECOVERY	CALORIES	PROTEIN (G)	FAT (G)	CARBS (G)	FIBER (G)	SODIUM (MG)
Pom Flax-tastic (p. 52)	319	5	9	58	6	141
Brocco Bana (p. 54)	511	8	6	119	16	24
Chia Charge (p. 56)	336	6	8	64	15	22
Orangavo (p. 58)*	823	17	27	134	14	53
Cherry Bomb (p. 60)	341	8	6	68	8	100
Grape Trifecta (p. 62)	471	11	16	80	3	111
Nut Better (p. 64)	712	16	37	92	13	479
Pink Basil (p. 66)	425	14	19	80	10	120
Green Peach (p. 68)	117	3	<1	29	3	33
Mango-Yo (p. 70)	202	6	2	44	3	59
Kale Kiwi Tea (p. 72)	204	3	1	52	8	4
Sweet-Kea (p. 74)	246	6	2	52	5	52
Almond Joy (p. 76)	308	28	9	58	10	191
Raspberry Date (p. 78)	485	14	14	102	17	277
Cacao Delight (p. 80)	510	8	18	90	9	190
Tropical Turmeric (p. 82)	360	2	15	59	12	30
Green Monster (p. 84)	194	1	<1	49	7	39
Pollen Berry (p. 86)	427	7	18	69	15	193

*Given the calorie load, this smoothie can yield two servings.

POM FLAX-TASTIC

Serves: 1 | *Preparation: 5 minutes*

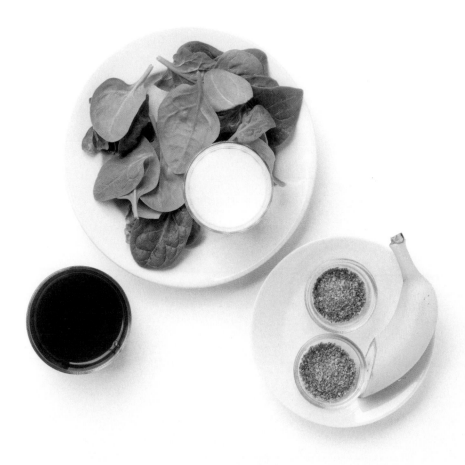

YOU NEED

1 cup rice milk • ½ cup pomegranate juice
a handful of baby spinach leaves • ½ banana, peeled and chopped
2 tablespoons ground flaxseed

Pomegranate juice is packed with powerful antioxidants,
which can lead to better heart health.

A *Anti-inflammatory*   **V** *Vitamin boosting*   **M** *Mineral enriching*

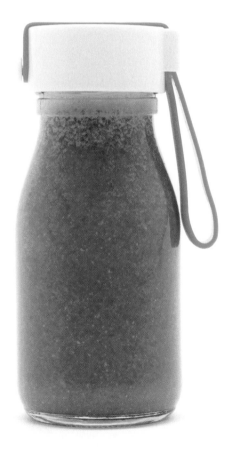

Place all the ingredients in a blender and blend until smooth.

BROCCO BANA

Serves: 1 | Preparation: 5 minutes

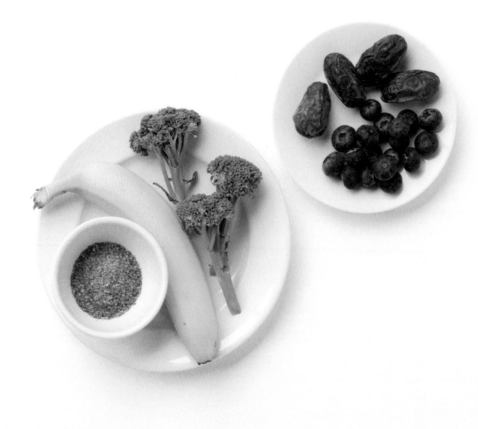

YOU NEED

1 banana, peeled and chopped • ⅔ cup broccoli florets • ½ cup blueberries
4 Medjool dates, pitted • 2 tablespoons ground flaxseed

Broccoli contains high levels of calcium and vitamin K,
both of which are important for bone health.

I *Immunity boosting* **B** *Brain boosting* **D** *Aids digestion*

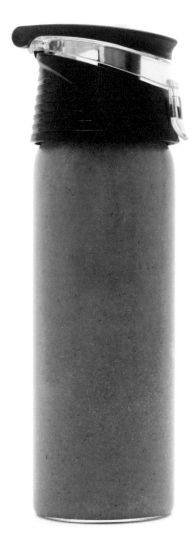

Place all the ingredients in a blender with 1 cup water and blend until smooth.

CHIA CHARGE

Serves: 1 | *Preparation: 5 minutes*

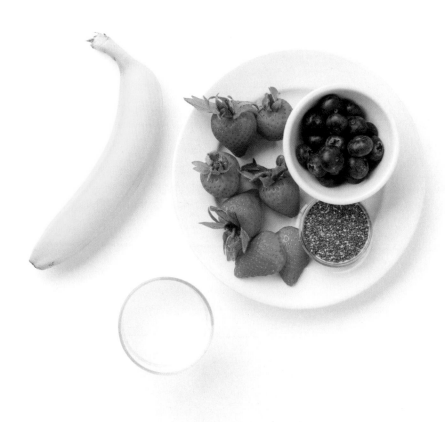

YOU NEED

1 cup coconut water • 1 banana, peeled and chopped
½ cup strawberries, hulled • ⅓ cup blueberries • 2 tablespoons chia seeds

Chia seeds are loaded with fiber, protein, omega-3 fatty acids, and various other micronutrients.

E *Energy boosting* **B** *Bone strengthening* **M** *Mineral enriching*

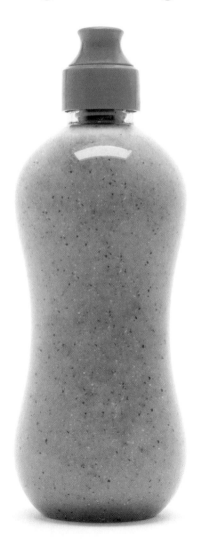

Place all the ingredients in a blender with ½ cup water and blend until smooth.

ORANGAVO

Serves: 1–2 | Preparation: 5 minutes

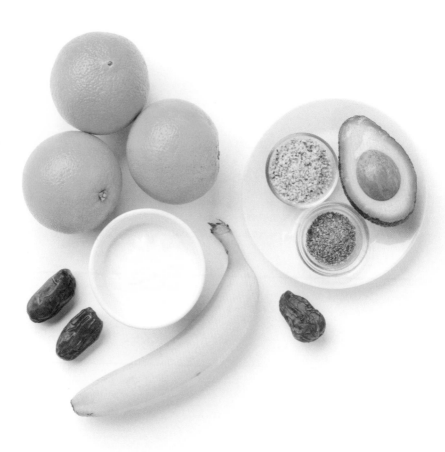

YOU NEED

juice of 3 oranges • ½ avocado, pitted and peeled
1 banana, peeled and chopped • ¼ cup plain yogurt
2 tablespoons shelled hemp seeds • 1 tablespoon ground flaxseed
3 Medjool dates, pitted

Avocado, flaxseed, and hemp seeds all contain fatty acids, which promote healthy brain function.

S *Skin enhancing* **P** *Protein boosting* **V** *Vitamin boosting*

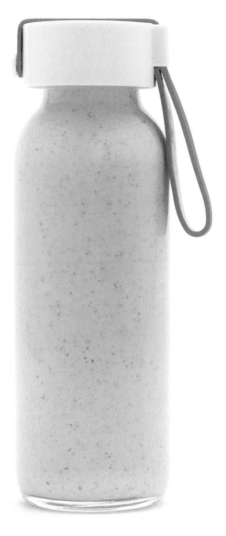

Place all the ingredients in a blender and blend until smooth. Add some water to loosen the mixture if you prefer.

CHERRY BOMB

Serves: 1 | Preparation: 5 minutes

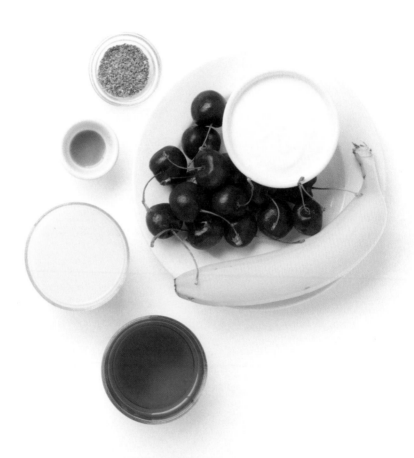

YOU NEED

¼ cup cherry juice • 1 cup oat milk • ⅓ cup plain yogurt
⅔ cup pitted cherries (fresh or frozen) • 1 banana, peeled and chopped
1 teaspoon pure vanilla extract • 1 tablespoon ground flaxseed

Cherry juice is high in antioxidants, which help reduce inflammation.

V *Vitamin boosting* **D** *Aids digestion* **M** *Mineral enriching*

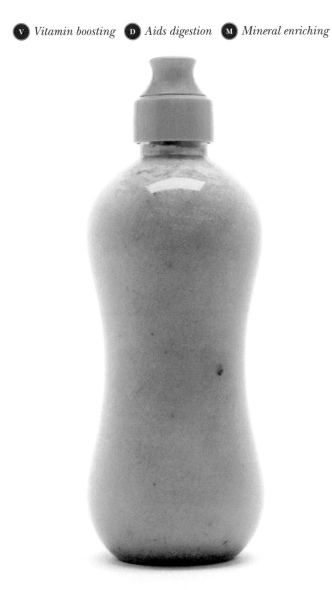

Place all the ingredients in a blender and blend until smooth.

GRAPE TRIFECTA

Serves: 1 | Preparation: 5 minutes

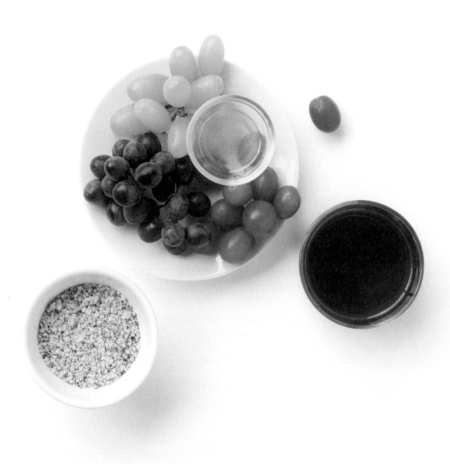

YOU NEED
1 cup grape juice • ½ cup red grapes • ½ cup black grapes
½ cup green grapes • juice of ¼ lemon • 3 tablespoons shelled hemp seeds

Grapes offer a host of benefits, namely quick energy
and antioxidants like vitamins A and C.

V *Vitamin boosting* **A** *Alkalizing* **I** *Immunity boosting*

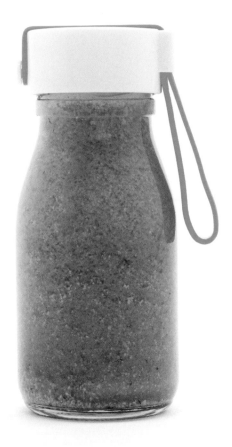

Place all the ingredients in a blender and blend until smooth.

NUT BETTER

Serves: 1 | Preparation: 5 minutes

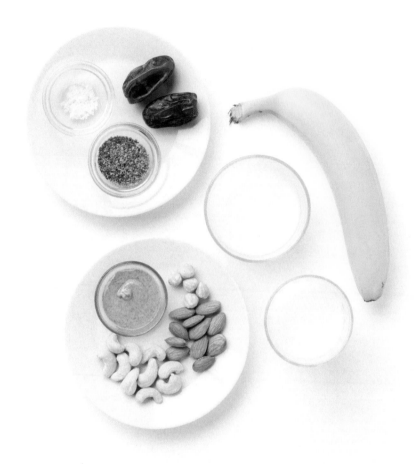

YOU NEED

1 cup almond milk • ½ cup coconut water • 10 raw almonds
10 raw cashew nuts • 5 raw hazelnuts, shelled • 1 banana, peeled and chopped
2 Medjool dates, pitted • 1 tablespoon smooth natural peanut butter
1 tablespoon ground flaxseed • a pinch of sea salt

Nuts are full of healthy fats, fiber, protein, magnesium, and vitamin E.

P *Protein boosting*   **D** *Aids digestion*   **I** *Immunity boosting*

Place all the ingredients in a blender and blend until smooth.

PINK BASIL

Serves: 1 | Preparation: 5 minutes

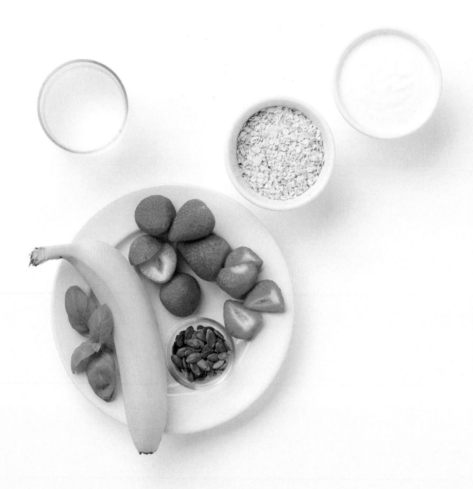

YOU NEED

1 cup coconut water • 1 banana, peeled and chopped
1 cup strawberries, halved • ½ cup plain yogurt
⅓ cup rolled oats • 1 tablespoon pumpkin seeds • 4 basil leaves

Basil contains antibacterial properties, which can boost immunity.

H *Hydrating*   **D** *Aids digestion*   **P** *Protein boosting*

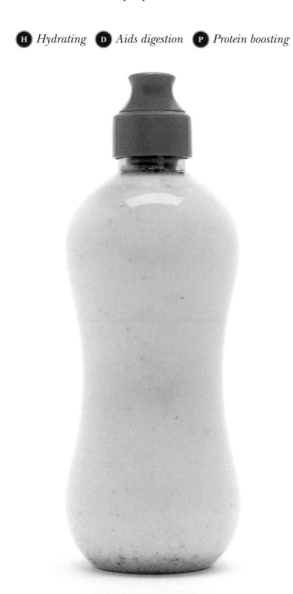

Place all the ingredients in a blender and blend until smooth.

GREEN PEACH

Serves: 1 | Preparation: 5 minutes

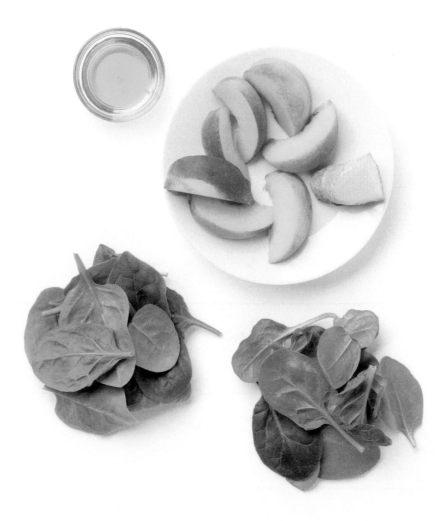

YOU NEED

2 handfuls of baby spinach • 1-inch piece of ginger, peeled
1 cup peach slices (fresh or frozen) • 2 teaspoons raw honey

Rich in B vitamins and electrolytes, this smoothie has the nutrients necessary to keep your cells and nerves in strong working order.

B *Bone strengthening*　**B** *Blood stimulating*　**I** *Immunity boosting*

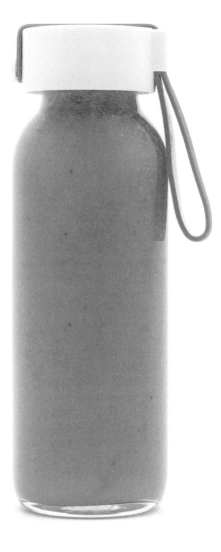

Place all the ingredients in a blender with 1 cup water and blend until smooth.

MANGO-YO

Serves: 1 | Preparation: 5 minutes

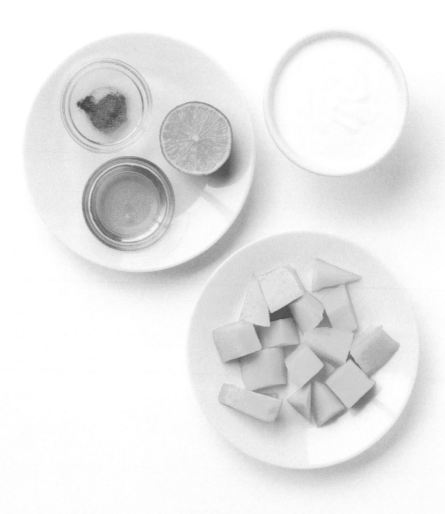

YOU NEED

1 cup mango chunks • ⅓ cup plain yogurt
½ teaspoon ground cinnamon • 1 tablespoon raw honey • juice of ½ lime

Mangoes are a great source of the flavonoid quercetin, which can help reduce inflammation.

V *Vitamin boosting* **D** *Aids digestion* **M** *Mineral enriching*

Place all the ingredients in a blender with 1 cup water and blend until smooth.

KALE KIWI TEA

Serves: 1 | Preparation: 5 minutes

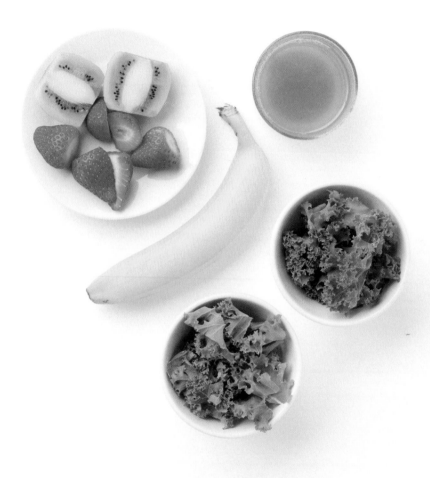

YOU NEED

1 cup green tea, chilled • 1 banana, peeled and chopped
2 handfuls of chopped kale • 1 kiwi, peeled and halved
4 strawberries, halved

Kiwis are packed full of vitamins C, K, and potassium.

B *Blood stimulating*   **E** *Energy boosting*   **V** *Vitamin boosting*

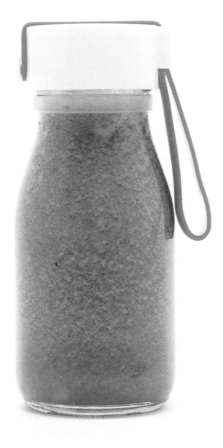

Place all the ingredients in a blender and blend until smooth.

SWEET-KEA

Serves: 1 | Preparation: 5 minutes

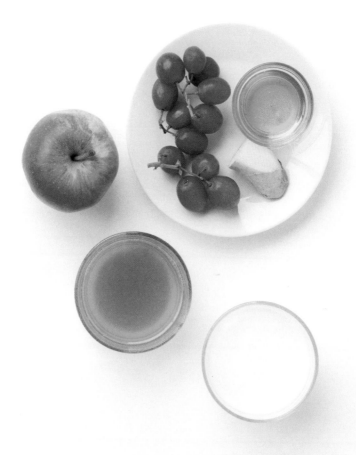

YOU NEED

½ cup green tea, chilled • 1 apple, cored • ½ cup red grapes
½ cup low-fat kefir milk • 1-inch piece of ginger, peeled
1 tablespoon raw honey

Kefir is high in nutrients and probiotics
and is beneficial for digestion and gut health.

D *Aids digestion* **I** *Immunity boosting* **V** *Vitamin boosting*

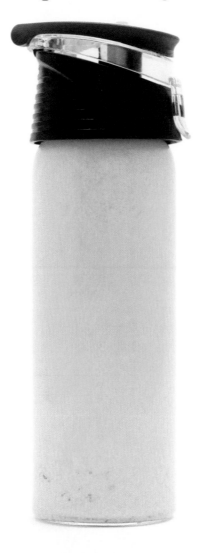

Place all the ingredients in a blender with ⅓ cup water and blend until smooth.

ALMOND JOY

Serves: 1 | Preparation: 5 minutes

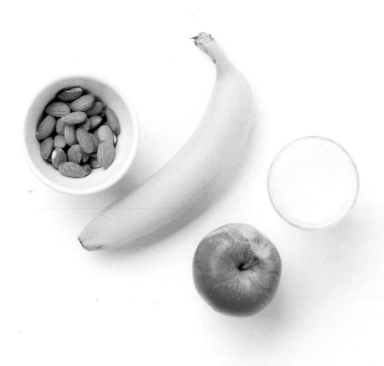

YOU NEED

1 cup almond milk • 1 banana, peeled and chopped
1 apple, cored • 2 tablespoons raw almonds

Almonds are beneficial for heart health, and fortified almond milk is rich in calcium and protein—just check the label.

P *Protein boosting*　　**M** *Mineral enriching*　　**V** *Vitamin boosting*

Place all the ingredients in a blender and blend until smooth.

RASPBERRY DATE

Serves: 1 | Preparation: 5 minutes

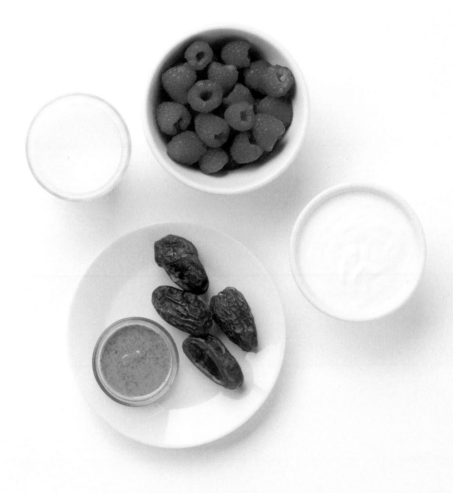

YOU NEED

1 cup almond milk • 1 cup raspberries • ½ cup plain yogurt
4 Medjool dates, pitted • 1 tablespoon smooth natural almond butter

Raspberries are low in calories and saturated fats,
but are a rich source of dietary fiber and antioxidants.

I *Immunity boosting*   **D** *Aids digestion*   **E** *Energy boosting*

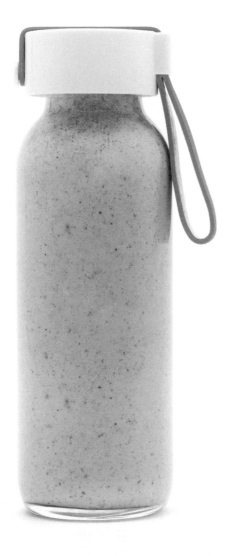

Place all the ingredients in a blender and blend until smooth.

CACAO DELIGHT

Serves: 1 | Preparation: 5 minutes

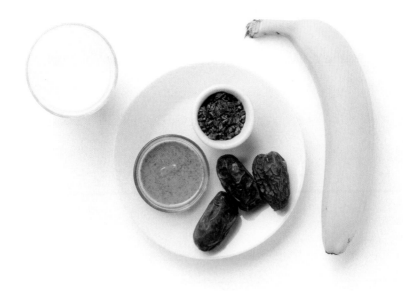

YOU NEED

1 cup almond milk • 1 banana, peeled and chopped
1 tablespoon smooth natural almond butter • 3 Medjool dates, pitted
1 tablespoon cacao nibs

Cacao is among the highest plant-based sources of iron.

B *Blood stimulating*   **P** *Protein boosting*   **S** *Skin enhancing*

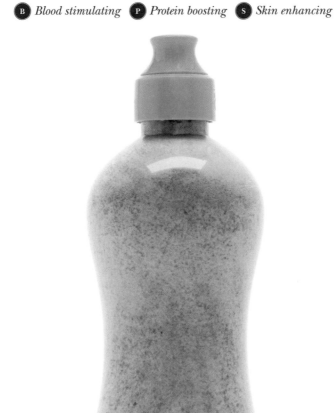

Place all the ingredients in a blender and blend until smooth.

TROPICAL TURMERIC

Serves: 1 | Preparation: 5 minutes

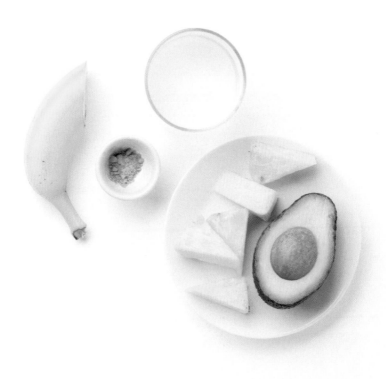

YOU NEED

1 cup coconut water • 1 cup pineapple chunks
½ banana, peeled and chopped • ½ avocado, pitted and peeled
½ teaspoon ground turmeric

Turmeric contains curcumin, which is a natural anti-inflammatory.

S *Skin enhancing* **V** *Vitamin boosting* **I** *Immunity boosting*

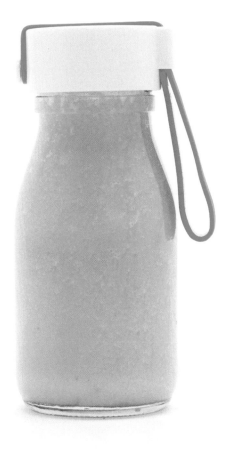

Place all the ingredients in a blender and blend until smooth.

GREEN MONSTER

Serves: 1 | Preparation: 5 minutes

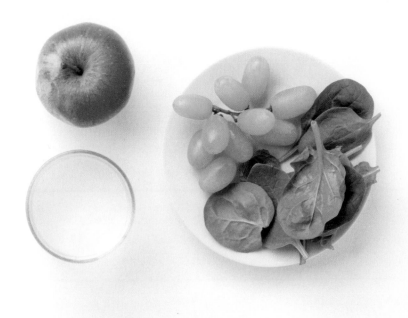

YOU NEED

1 cup coconut water • a handful of baby spinach leaves
10 green grapes (fresh or frozen) • 1 apple, cored

Coconut water is rich in potassium,
which helps balance the sodium in a healthy diet.

M *Mineral boosting* **B** *Brain boosting* **H** *Hydrating*

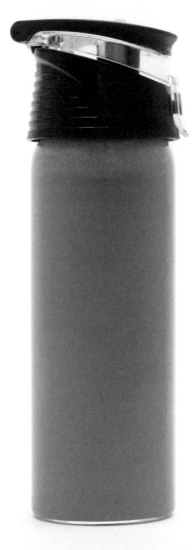

Place all the ingredients in a blender and blend until smooth.

POLLEN BERRY

Serves: 1 | Preparation: 5 minutes

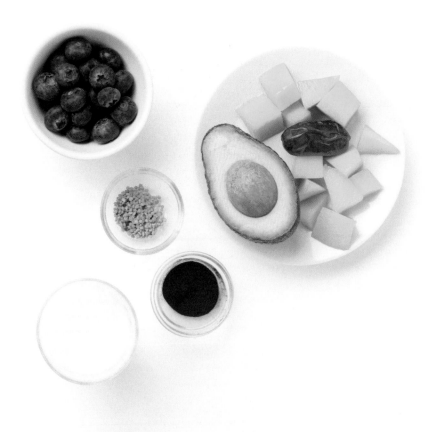

YOU NEED

1 cup almond milk • 1 cup blueberries
⅔ cup mango chunks • 1 teaspoon bee pollen • 1 Medjool date, pitted
½ avocado, pitted and peeled • 1 teaspoon spirulina powder

Bee pollen is 20 percent protein and rich in nutrients. Spirulina and berries round out this nutritional powerhouse.

(S) *Skin enhancing*   **(P)** *Protein boosting*   **(V)** *Vitamin boosting*

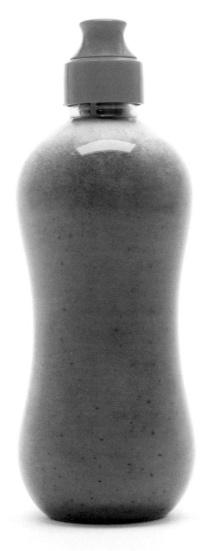

Place all the ingredients in a blender and blend until smooth.

MUSCLE-BUILDING

*Whether you have a regular routine
of weight-lifting at the gym or making time
for strength-building in the off-season,
it's helpful to tip your macronutrient
balance to include more protein to
complement your goals. These smoothies are
best consumed at the end of your workout.*

MUSCLE-BUILDING SMOOTHIES	CALORIES	PROTEIN (G)	FAT (G)	CARBS (G)	FIBER (G)	SODIUM (MG)
Oat & Tofu (p. 90)	363	12	21	37	10	198
Coco Melon (p. 92)	321	15	11	44	3	175
Magic Mango (p. 94)	392	6	12	68	9	33
Fruity Kale (p. 96)	474	11	4	110	17	127
Papaya Passion (p. 98)	245	10	9	36	10	190
Kiwi Raspberry (p. 100)	274	9	7	72	9	96
Oaty Apple (p. 102)	347	8	14	50	10	37
Caribbean Kick (p. 104)	485	11	27	59	15	207
Green Protein (p. 106)	340	26	11	37	9	384
Loca Mocha (p. 108)	306	9	17	33	6	162
Cranberry Pro (p. 110)	388	9	19	50	9	36
Blue Cashew (p. 112)	396	27	13	47	8	401
Pumpkin Patch (p. 114)	347	31	13	32	9	337
Banana Nut (p. 116)	340	26	11	38	7	350
Super Goji (p. 118)	227	16	7	41	5	159
Piña Spirulina (p. 120)	242	4	5	51	6	55
Peanut Chia (p. 122)	512	8	12	106	10	144

OAT & TOFU

Serves: 1 | Preparation: 5 minutes

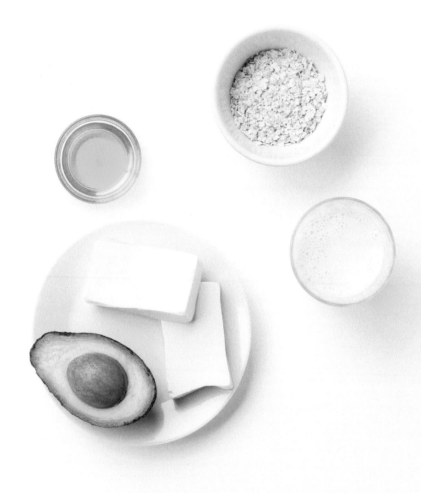

YOU NEED

1 cup almond milk • ¼ cup rolled oats • ⅔ cup firm silken tofu
1 tablespoon raw honey • ½ avocado, pitted and peeled

Tofu is an excellent source of amino acids.

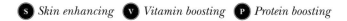 **S** *Skin enhancing* **V** *Vitamin boosting* **P** *Protein boosting*

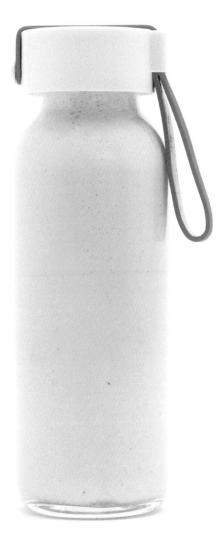

Place all the ingredients in a blender and blend until smooth.

COCO MELON

Serves: 1 | Preparation: 5 minutes

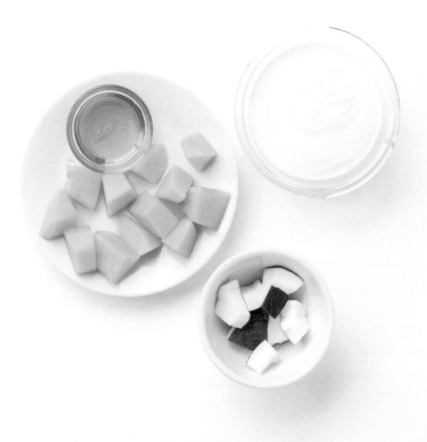

YOU NEED

1 cup cantaloupe, peeled, seeded, and cut into chunks
¼ cup coconut meat • 1 cup plain yogurt • 1 tablespoon raw honey

Cantaloupe is a rehydration and immunity powerhouse, packing in electrolytes like potassium and vitamin C.

D *Aids digestion* **H** *Hydrating* **V** *Vitamin boosting*

Place all the ingredients in a blender and blend until smooth.

MAGIC MANGO

Serves: 1 | Preparation: 5 minutes

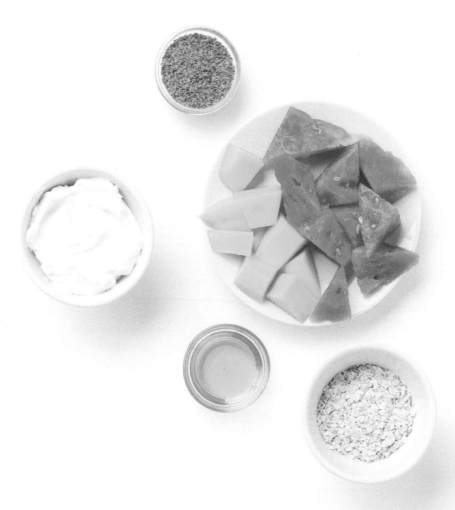

YOU NEED

1 cup watermelon, peeled, seeded, and cut into chunks
½ cup mango chunks • ½ cup coconut yogurt • 3 tablespoons rolled oats
2 tablespoons ground flaxseed • 1 teaspoon raw honey

Watermelon has high levels of lycopene, which is very effective
at protecting cells from damage.

M *Mineral boosting* **H** *Hydrating* **D** *Aids digestion*

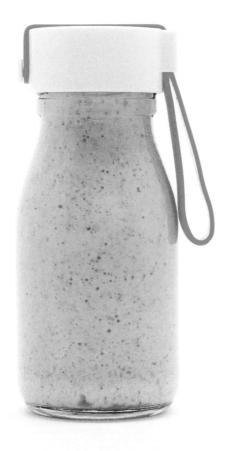

Place all the ingredients in a blender with ½ cup water and blend until smooth.

FRUITY KALE

Serves: 1 | Preparation: 5 minutes

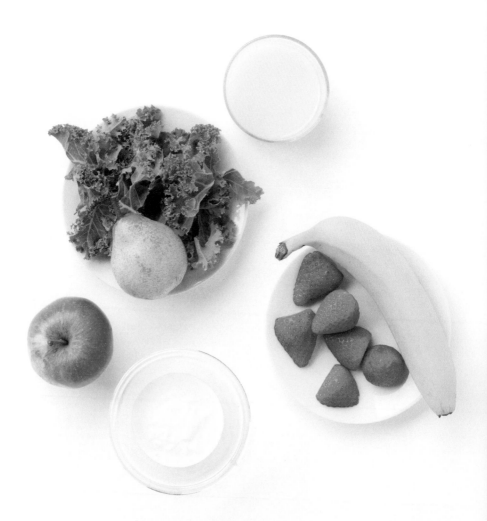

YOU NEED

⅔ cup oat milk • ½ cup chopped kale • 1 banana, peeled and chopped
1 apple, cored • 6 strawberries, hulled • 1 pear, cored • ¼ cup plain yogurt

Kale is rich in vitamin A, which helps keep the eyes healthy.

I *Immunity boosting*   **E** *Energy boosting*   **B** *Bone strengthening*

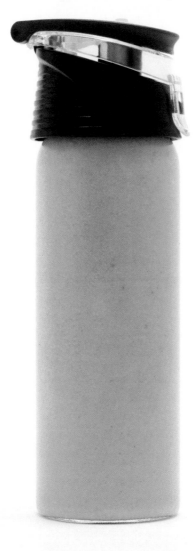

Place all the ingredients in a blender and blend until smooth.

PAPAYA PASSION

Serves: 1 | Preparation: 5 minutes

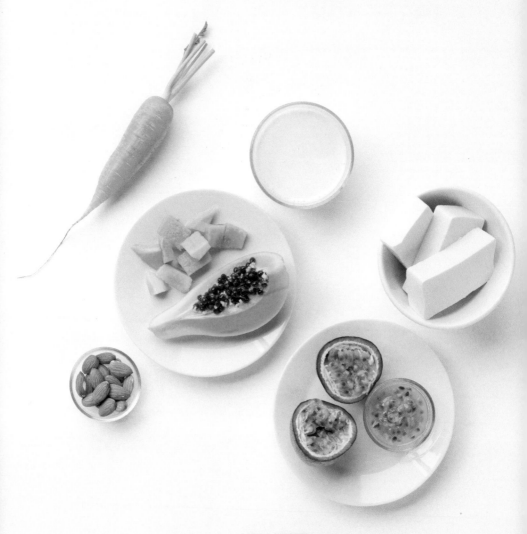

YOU NEED

1 cup almond milk • ½ cup papaya, peeled, seeded, and chopped
2 passion fruit, pulp only • 1 carrot, peeled • ⅔ cup firm silken tofu
1 tablespoon raw almonds

Rich in vitamin C and iron, this smoothie serves up
two essential nutrients that rely on each other for absorbtion.

D *Aids digestion* **V** *Vitamin boosting* **P** *Protein boosting*

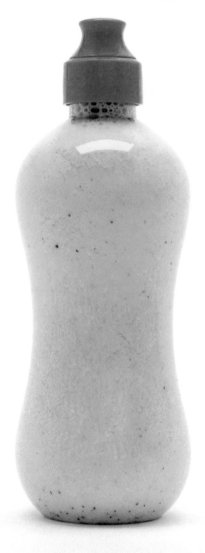

Place all the ingredients in a blender and blend until smooth.

KIWI RASPBERRY

Serves: 1 | Preparation: 5 minutes

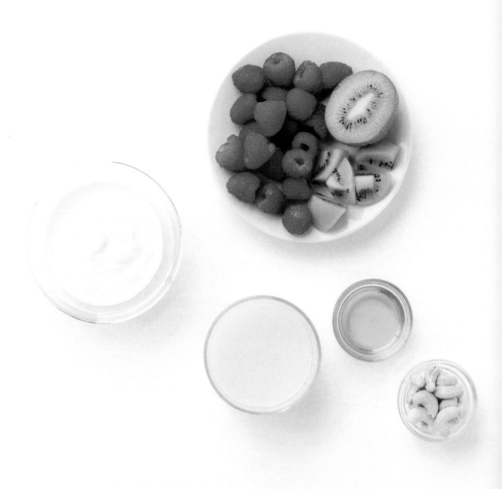

YOU NEED

½ cup oat milk • ¾ cup raspberries • 1 kiwi, peeled
⅓ cup plain yogurt • 1 teaspoon raw honey • 1 tablespoon raw cashew nuts

Raspberries are packed with vitamin C, which is necessary for growth and repair of cells in the body.

(V) *Vitamin boosting*   (D) *Aids digestion*   (P) *Protein boosting*

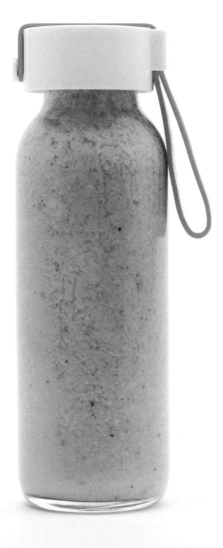

Place all the ingredients in a blender and blend until smooth.

OATY APPLE

Serves: 1 | Preparation: 5 minutes

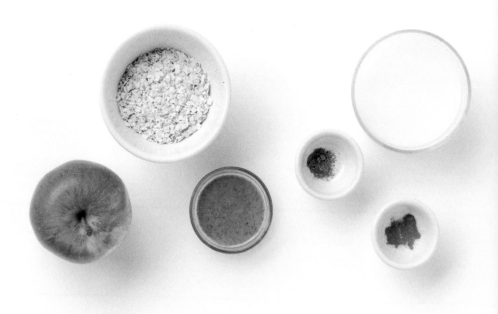

YOU NEED

½ cup unsweetened coconut milk • 1 apple, cored
¼ cup rolled oats • ½ teaspoon ground cinnamon
½ teaspoon ground nutmeg • 1 tablespoon natural smooth almond butter

Apples are high in potassium—a vital mineral for healthy blood pressure.

P *Protein boosting* **V** *Vitamin boosting* **D** *Aids digestion*

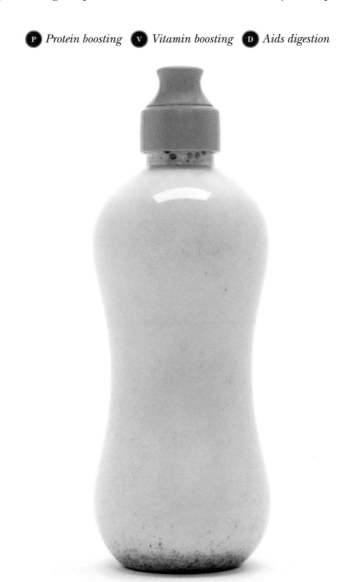

Place all the ingredients in a blender with ½ cup water and blend until smooth.

CARIBBEAN KICK

Serves: 1 | *Preparation: 5 minutes*

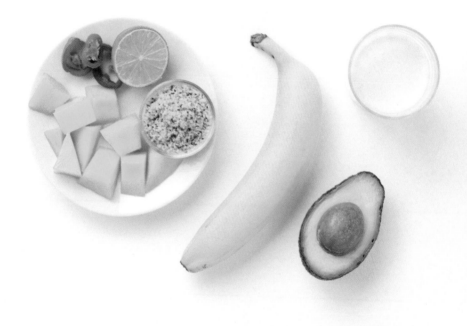

YOU NEED

1 cup almond milk • 1 banana, peeled and chopped • ⅔ cup mango chunks
3 slices pickled jalepeño • ½ avocado, pitted and peeled
2 tablespoons shelled hemp seeds • juice of ½ lime

Mangoes are high in potassium and contain good amounts of calcium, iron, magnesium, and phosphorus.

P *Protein boosting* **S** *Skin enhancing* **V** *Vitamin boosting*

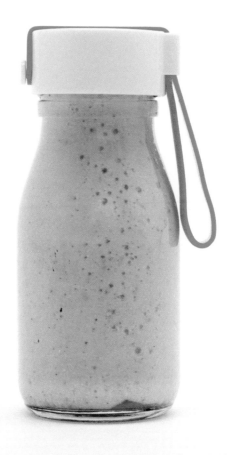

Place all the ingredients in a blender and blend until smooth.

GREEN PROTEIN

Serves: 1 | Preparation: 5 minutes

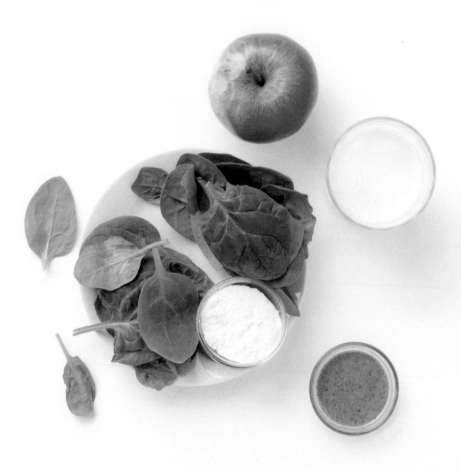

YOU NEED

1 cup almond milk • 1 apple, cored • 2 handfuls of baby spinach leaves
1 tablespoon natural smooth almond butter • 1 scoop protein powder

Spinach is a great source of iron, niacin, and zinc.
It also contains vitamins A, C, E, B6, and K.

P *Protein boosting*   **D** *Aids digestion*   **E** *Energy boosting*

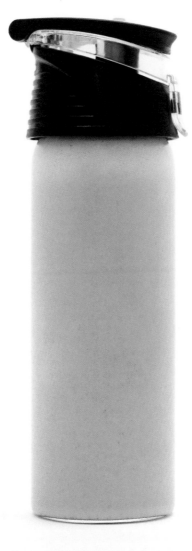

Place all the ingredients in a blender and blend until smooth.

LOCA MOCHA

Serves: 1 | Preparation: 5 minutes

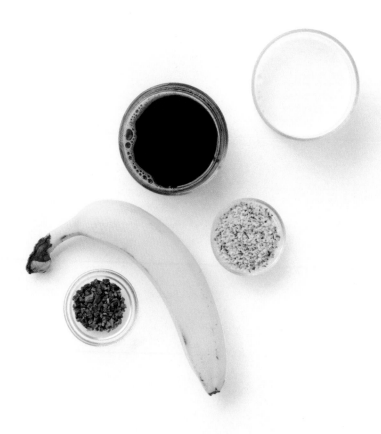

YOU NEED

1 cup cashew milk • 1 banana, peeled and chopped
½ cup filtered coffee, chilled • 2 tablespoons shelled hemp seeds
1 tablespoon cacao nibs

Cashew milk is a good source of fiber and vitamin E.

E *Energy boosting*　　**P** *Protein boosting*　　**B** *Bone strengthening*

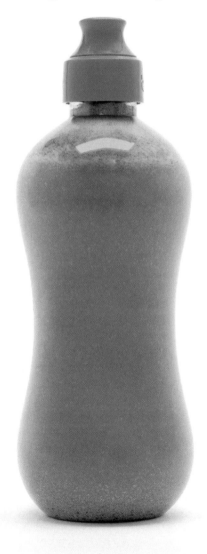

Place all the ingredients in a blender and blend until smooth.

CRANBERRY PRO

Serves: 1 | Preparation: 5 minutes

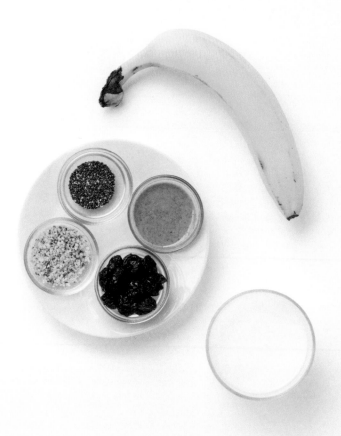

YOU NEED

1 cup unsweetened coconut milk • 1 banana, peeled and chopped
2 tablespoons dried cranberries • 1 tablespoon natural smooth almond butter
1 tablespoon shelled hemp seeds • ½ tablespoon chia seeds

Cranberries contain proanthocyanidins, antioxidants known to fight infection, stomach ulcers, and even dental issues.

P *Protein boosting* **M** *Mineral enriching* **B** *Bone strengthening*

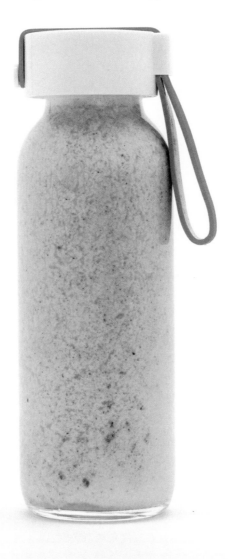

Place all the ingredients in a blender and blend until smooth.

BLUE CASHEW

Serves: 1 | Preparation: 5 minutes

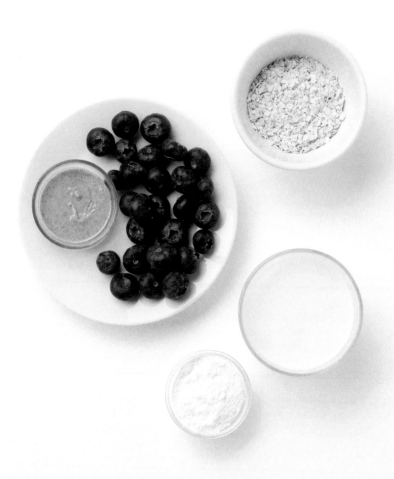

YOU NEED

1 cup cashew milk • ¼ cup rolled oats • 1 cup blueberries
1 scoop protein powder • 1 tablespoon natural cashew nut butter

Blueberries may help with blood sugar regulation.

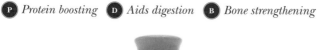 **P** *Protein boosting* **D** *Aids digestion* **B** *Bone strengthening*

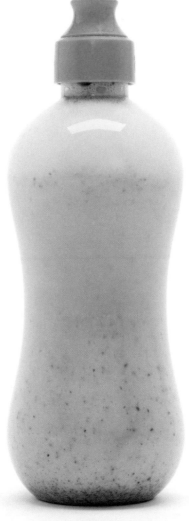

Place all the ingredients in a blender and blend until smooth.

PUMPKIN PATCH

Serves: 1 | Preparation: 5 minutes

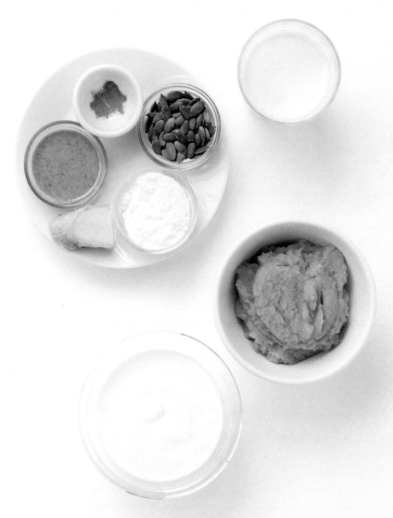

YOU NEED

¾ cup pumpkin purée • 1 tablespoon natural smooth almond butter
1 scoop protein powder • ⅓ cup plain yogurt • ½ cup almond milk
1-inch piece of ginger, peeled • a pinch of ground cinnamon
1 teaspoon pumpkin seeds

This smoothie is high in fiber and contains probiotics,
both of which help with digestion.

B *Blood stimulating* **A** *Anti-inflammatory* **P** *Protein boosting*

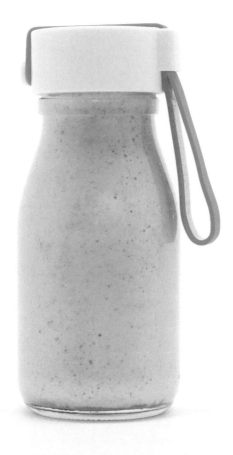

Place all the ingredients in a blender and blend until smooth.

BANANA NUT

Serves: 1 | Preparation: 5 minutes

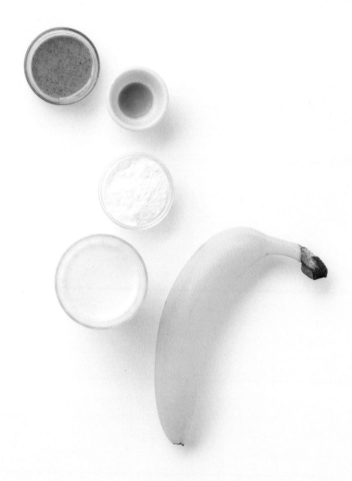

YOU NEED

1 cup almond milk • 1 banana, peeled and chopped
1 tablespoon natural smooth almond butter • 1 scoop protein powder
1 teaspoon pure vanilla extract

Bananas are packed with potassium,
which keeps energy stores flowing throughout the body.

I *Immunity boosting*   **P** *Protein boosting*   **B** *Bone strengthening*

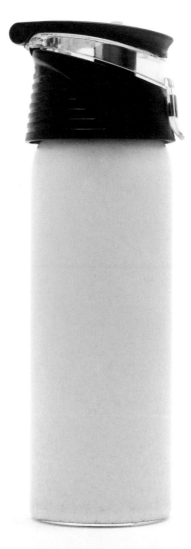

Place all the ingredients in a blender and blend until smooth.

SUPER GOJI

Serves: 1 | Preparation: 5 minutes

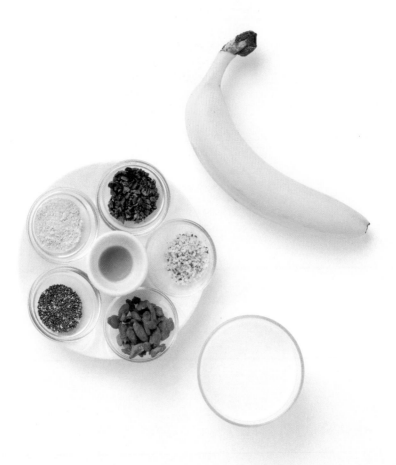

YOU NEED

1 cup cashew milk • 1 banana, peeled and chopped
1 teaspoon maca powder • 1 teaspoon chia seeds
1 teaspoon shelled hemp seeds • ½ teaspoon pure vanilla extract
1 teaspoon goji berries • 1 teaspoon cacao nibs

Goji berries are full of nutrients that benefit heart health and circulation.

V *Vitamin boosting* **E** *Energy boosting* **M** *Mineral enriching*

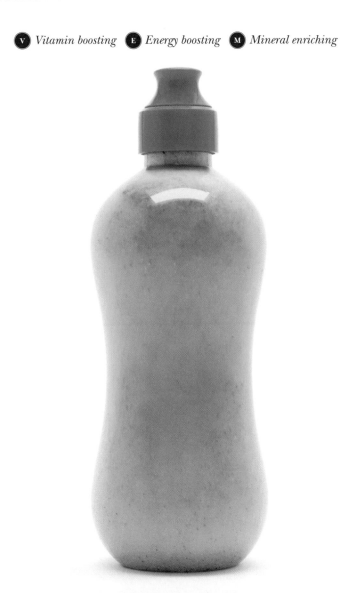

Place all the ingredients in a blender and blend until smooth.

PIÑA SPIRULINA

Serves: 1 | Preparation: 5 minutes

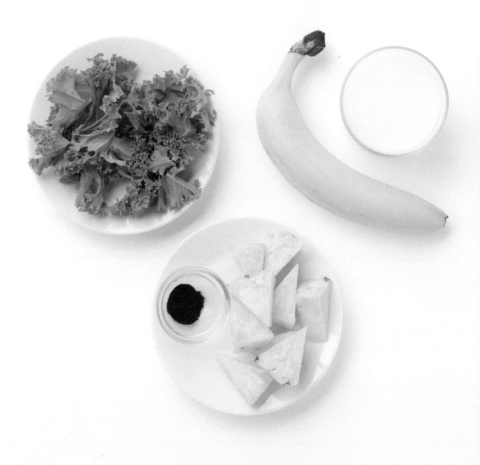

YOU NEED

1 cup unsweetened coconut milk • a handful of chopped kale
1 cup pineapple chunks • 1 banana, peeled and chopped
½ teaspoon spirulina powder

Spirulina is more than 70 percent protein and
packed full of vitamins and minerals.

(A) *Anti-inflammatory*   **(E)** *Energy boosting*   **(M)** *Mineral enriching*

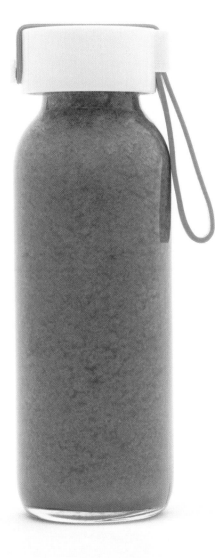

Place all the ingredients in a blender and blend until smooth.

PEANUT CHIA

Serves: 1 | Preparation: 5 minutes

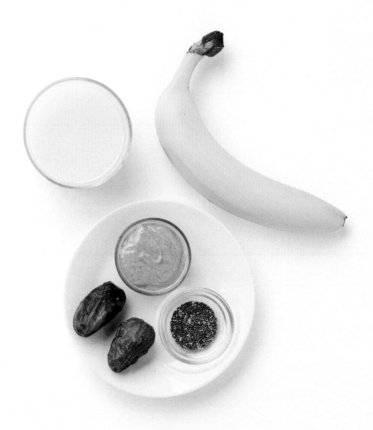

YOU NEED

½ cup rice milk • 1 banana, peeled and chopped
1 heaped tablespoon natural smooth peanut butter
2 Medjool dates, pitted • 1 teaspoon chia seeds

Peanuts are a good source of protein and are packed with healthy fat.

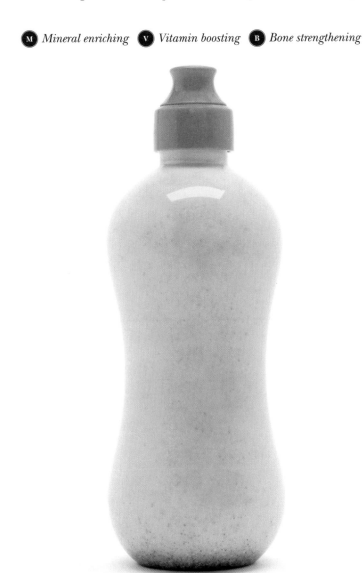 **M** *Mineral enriching*   **V** *Vitamin boosting*   **B** *Bone strengthening*

Place all the ingredients in a blender with ½ cup water and blend until smooth.

CARB-LOADING

These are smoothies will build up your glycogen stores before a big effort or event. If you are running a marathon, doing a long bike ride or even a triathlon, you might find it hard to get in all of the carbs your body needs. These smoothies pack in the energy to help you do just that.

CARB-LOADING SMOOTHIES	CALORIES	PROTEIN (G)	FAT (G)	CARBS (G)	FIBER (G)	SODIUM (MG)
Peach Carbler (p. 126)	342	13	11	54	9	95
Cacao Flax (p. 128)	404	9	12	70	9	57
Sweet Potato Jive (p. 130)	347	5	3	79	6	94
Spinachia (p. 132)	444	29	16	51	12	237
Almond Load (p. 134)	218	6	7	38	7	176
Branberry Rocket (p. 136)	480	18	6	101	14	317
Back in Black (p. 138)	388	19	19	40	12	101
Nutty Boom (p. 140)	647	22	46	47	10	231
Orange Tornado (p. 142)	270	5	3	84	10	94
Peachellini (p. 144)	331	10	6	60	14	104
Oat Me Up (p. 146)	514	10	10	105	12	101
Sweet Papaya Poyo (p. 148)	394	18	7	71	7	116
Veggie Beet (p. 150)	280	4	4	63	8	169
Sweet Potana (p. 152)	538	9	21	82	8	95
Buckwheat Bang (p. 154)	463	16	7	60	9	117
Orangey Apricot (p. 156)	385	10	4	83	12	130

PEACH CARBLER

Serves: 1 | Preparation: 5 minutes

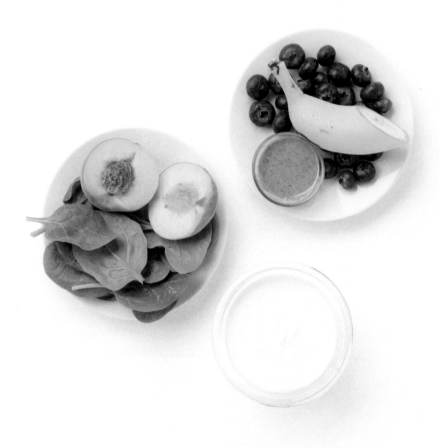

YOU NEED

½ cup plain yogurt • ½ banana, peeled and chopped
⅔ cup blueberries • 1 peach, halved and pitted
a handful of baby spinach leaves • 1 tablespoon natural smooth almond butter

Peaches are full of folic acid, potassium, and vitamins A, C, and E.

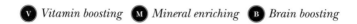 *Vitamin boosting* *Mineral enriching* *Brain boosting*

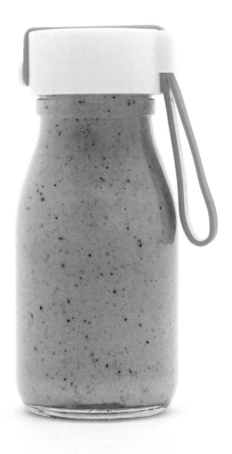

Place all the ingredients in a blender with ½ cup water
and blend until smooth.

CACAO FLAX

Serves: 1 | Preparation: 5 minutes

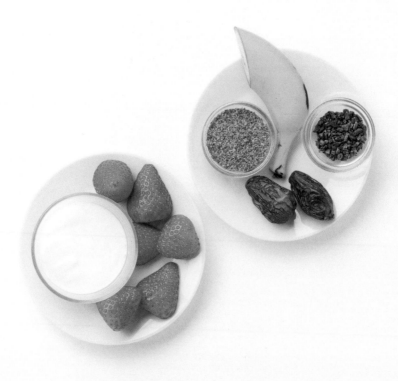

YOU NEED

½ cup strawberries, hulled • ½ banana, peeled and chopped
⅓ cup plain yogurt • 2 tablespoons ground flaxseed
1 tablespoon cacao nibs • 2 Medjool dates, pitted

Flaxseeds are a rich source of omega-3 fatty acids and fiber, nutrients that can lead to better heart health.

B *Blood stimulating*   **D** *Aids digestion*   **V** *Vitamin boosting*

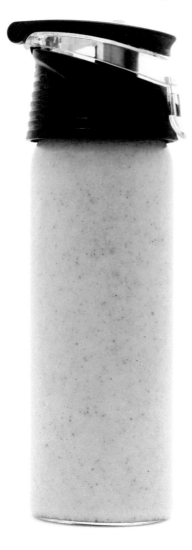

Place all the ingredients in a blender with ¾ cup water and blend until smooth.

SWEET POTATO JIVE

Serves: 1 | Preparation: 5 minutes

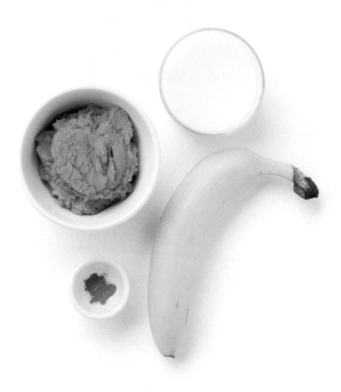

YOU NEED

1 cup rice milk • ½ cup sweet potato, cooked, cooled, and mashed
1 banana, peeled and chopped • a pinch of ground cinnamon

Sweet potatoes are high in vitamins A and C,
beta-carotene, and manganese.

I *Immunity boosting*   **M** *Mineral enriching*   **B** *Bone strengthening*

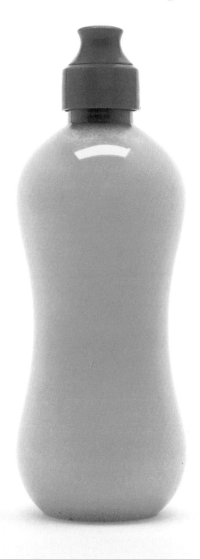

Place all the ingredients in a blender and blend until smooth.

SPINACHIA

Serves: 1 | *Preparation: 5 minutes*

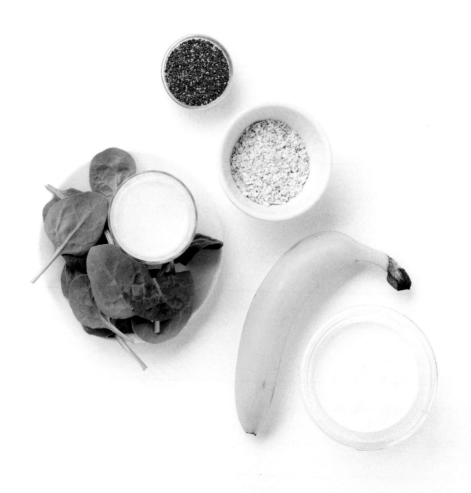

YOU NEED

½ cup almond milk • a handful of baby spinach leaves
1 cup plain Greek yogurt • 1 banana, peeled and chopped
2 tablespoons chia seeds • 2 tablespoons rolled oats

Greek yogurt is full of probiotics, which help regulate digestion.

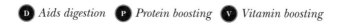 **D** *Aids digestion* **P** *Protein boosting* **V** *Vitamin boosting*

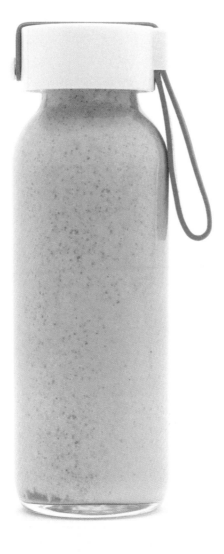

Place all the ingredients in a blender and blend until smooth.

ALMOND LOAD

Serves: 1 | *Preparation: 5 minutes*

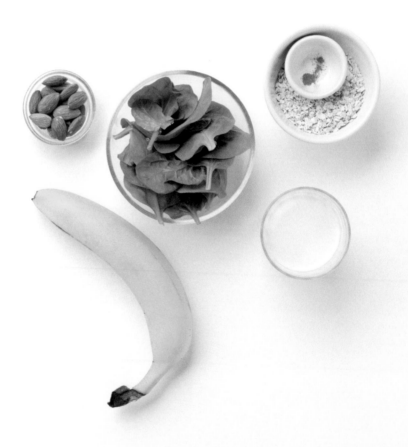

YOU NEED

1 cup almond milk • a handful of baby spinach leaves
2 tablespoons rolled oats • 1 banana, peeled and chopped
a pinch of ground cinnamon • 1 tablespoon raw almonds

Oats contain a powerful soluble fiber called beta-glucan,
which can help lower cholesterol.

Ⓜ *Mineral enriching* Ⓑ *Bone strengthening* Ⓔ *Energy boosting*

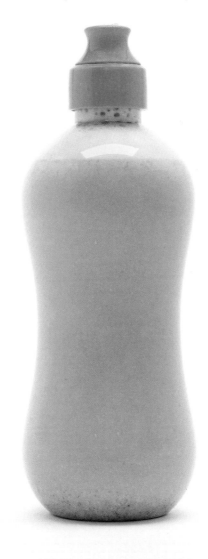

Place all the ingredients in a blender and blend until smooth.

BRANBERRY ROCKET

Serves: 1 | Preparation: 5 minutes

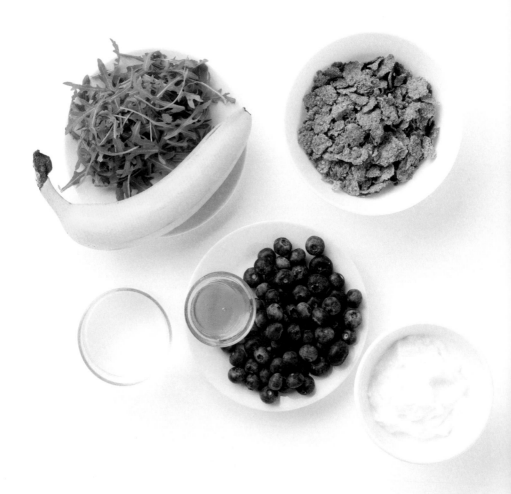

YOU NEED

1 cup bran flakes • 1 banana, peeled and chopped • ½ cup blueberries
a handful of arugula • ½ cup plain Greek yogurt • ¾ cup coconut water
1 tablespoon raw honey

Enriched bran flakes are high in fiber and
contain half of your daily iron needs.

D *Aids digestion*　**I** *Immunity boosting*　**V** *Vitamin boosting*

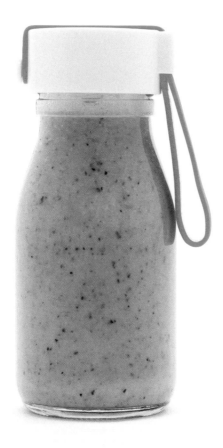

Place all the ingredients in a blender and blend until smooth.

BACK IN BLACK

Serves: 1 | Preparation: 5 minutes

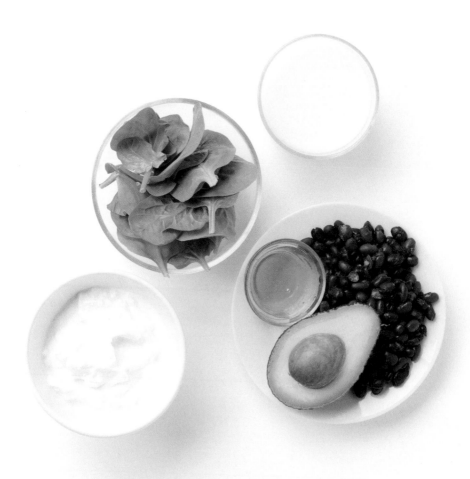

YOU NEED

⅓ cup cooked black beans, cooled • ⅔ cup rice milk
a handful of baby spinach leaves • ½ cup plain Greek yogurt
½ avocado, pitted and peeled • 1 tablespoon raw honey

Black beans are full of fiber, potassium, folate, and vitamin B6, which can help support heart health.

P *Protein boosting*   **S** *Skin enhancing*   **M** *Mineral enriching*

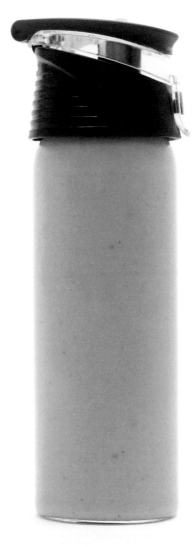

Place all the ingredients in a blender and blend until smooth.

NUTTY BOOM

Serves: 1 | Preparation: 5 minutes

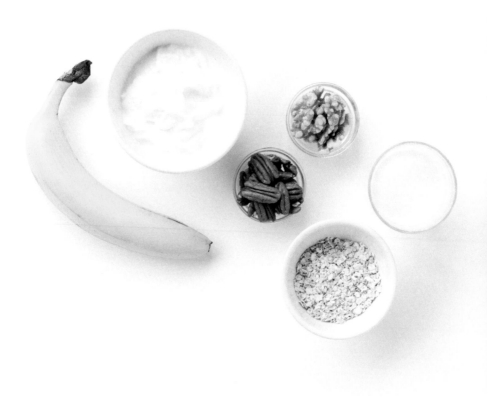

YOU NEED

½ cup almond milk • 1 banana, peeled and chopped
a small handful of walnuts • a small handful of pecans
½ cup plain Greek yogurt • 2 tablespoons rolled oats

Walnuts are rich in omega-3 fatty acids and are a good source of monounsaturated fatty acids, which benefit heart health.

E *Energy boosting*　**M** *Mineral enriching*　**B** *Bone strengthening*

Place all the ingredients in a blender and blend until smooth.

ORANGE TORNADO

Serves: 1 | Preparation: 5 minutes

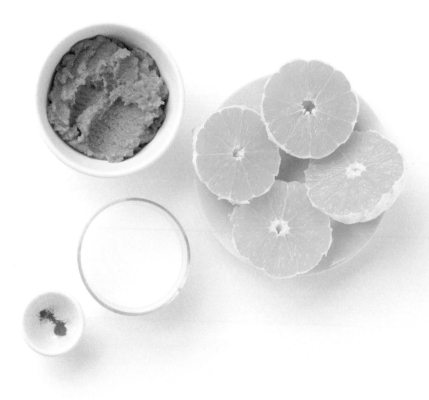

YOU NEED

1 cup rice milk • 1 cup sweet potato, cooked, cooled, and mashed
2 oranges, peeled and halved • a pinch of ground cinnamon

Oranges are high in vitamin C, which helps boost the immune system and helps fight skin damage from the sun.

V *Vitamin boosting*   **M** *Mineral enriching*   **E** *Energy boosting*

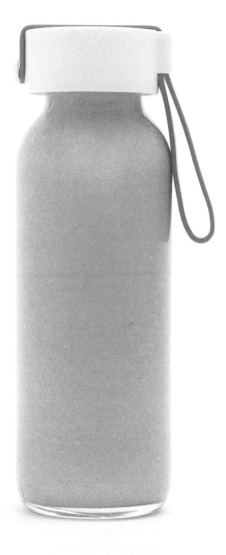

Place all the ingredients in a blender and blend until smooth.

PEACHELLINI

Serves: 1 | Preparation: 5 minutes

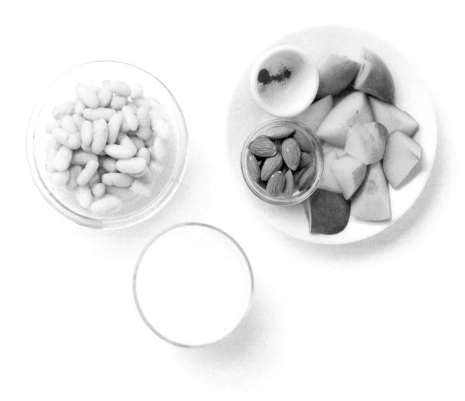

YOU NEED

⅔ cup cannellini beans, cooked and cooled
1 cup rice milk • 1 cup peach chunks
1 tablespoon raw almonds • a pinch of ground cinnamon

Cannellini beans are packed with antioxidants, iron, and dietary fiber.

P *Protein boosting*   **I** *Immunity boosting*   **V** *Vitamin boosting*

Place all the ingredients in a blender and blend until smooth.

OAT ME UP

Serves: 1 | Preparation: 5 minutes

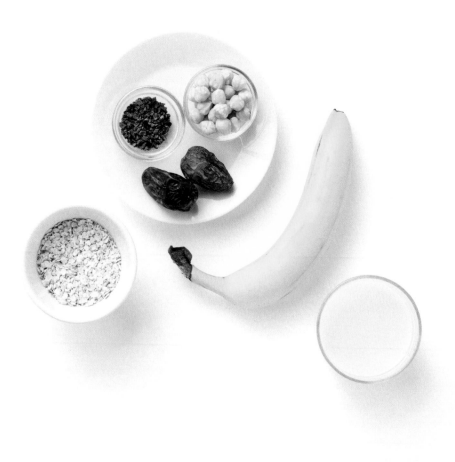

YOU NEED

1 cup oat milk • ¼ cup rolled oats • 1 banana, peeled and chopped
2 Medjool dates, pitted • 1 tablespoon raw blanched hazelnuts
1 teaspoon cacao nibs

Hazelnuts are full of vitamin E, which helps maintain healthy skin, hair, and nails.

P *Protein boosting*   **D** *Aids digestion*   **B** *Blood stimulating*

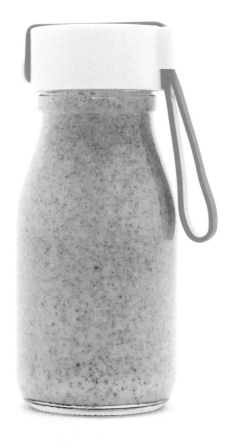

Place all the ingredients in a blender and blend until smooth.

SWEET PAPAYA POYO

Serves: 1 | Preparation: 5 minutes

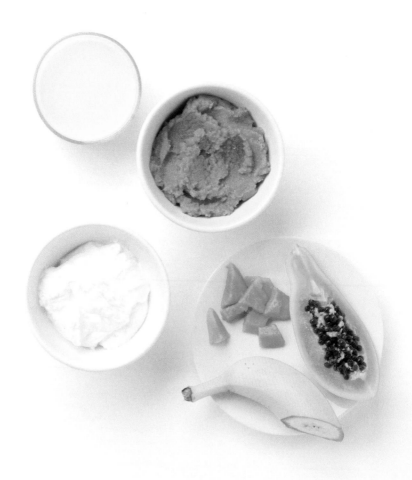

YOU NEED

1 cup sweet potato, cooked, cooled, and mashed • ½ cup plain Greek yogurt
½ cup soy milk • 1 small papaya, peeled, seeded, and cut into chunks
½ banana, peeled and chopped

Papaya is full of antioxidants, which can help reduce inflammation.

D *Aids digestion*   **S** *Skin enhancing*   **B** *Bone strengthening*

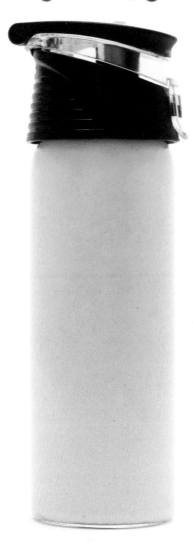

Place all the ingredients in a blender and blend until smooth.

VEGGIE BEET

Serves: 1 | Preparation: 5 minutes

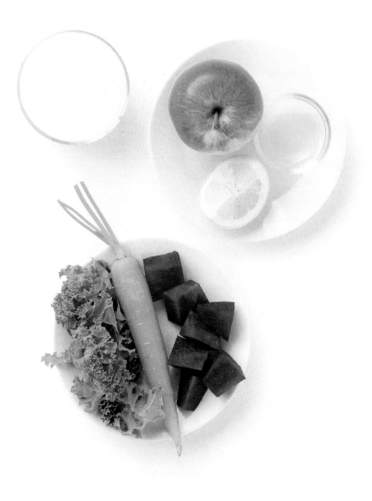

YOU NEED

1 cup rice milk • 1 small beet • 1 carrot, peeled
a handful of kale • juice of ½ lemon • 1 apple, cored

Beets are a good source of manganese, which helps with bone health and carbohydrate metabolism.

M *Mineral enriching*   **V** *Vitamin boosting*   **I** *Immunity boosting*

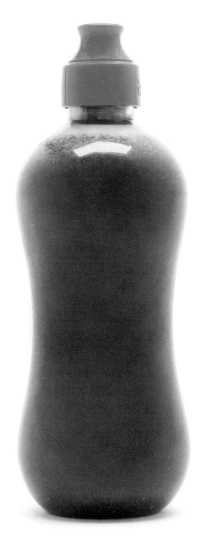

Place all the ingredients in a blender and blend until smooth.

SWEET POTANA

Serves: 1 | Preparation: 5 minutes

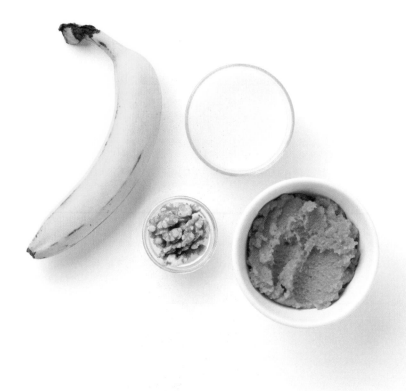

YOU NEED

1 cup sweet potato, cooked, cooled, and mashed • 1 cup rice milk
1 banana, peeled and chopped • a small handful of walnuts

Bananas have a high potassium content, which is necessary for good nerve and muscle function as well as maintaining a healthy balance of fluids in the body.

M *Mineral enriching* **S** *Skin enhancing* **P** *Protein boosting*

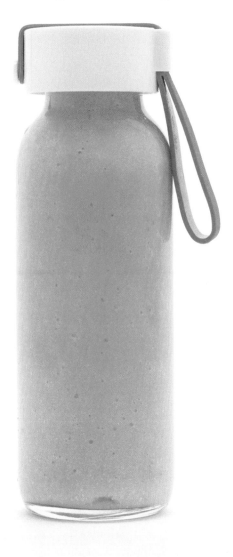

Place all the ingredients in a blender and blend until smooth.

BUCKWHEAT BANG

Serves: 1 | Preparation: 5 minutes

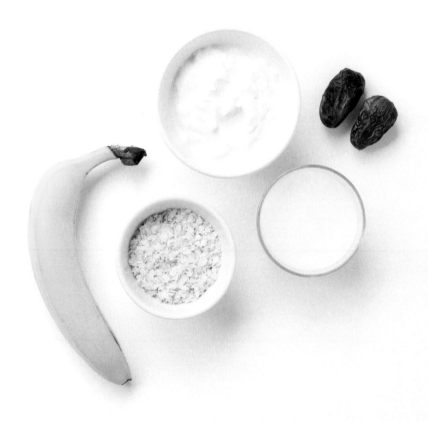

YOU NEED

2 tablespoons buckwheat flakes • ½ cup rice milk
⅓ cup plain Greek yogurt • 2 Medjool dates, pitted
1 banana, peeled and chopped

Buckwheat is full of nutrients and fiber, which can help control blood sugar levels, lowering blood glucose and insulin responses in the body.

D *Aids digestion*   **P** *Protein boosting*   **B** *Bone strengthening*

Place all the ingredients in a blender and blend until smooth.

ORANGEY APRICOT

Serves: 1 | Preparation: 5 minutes

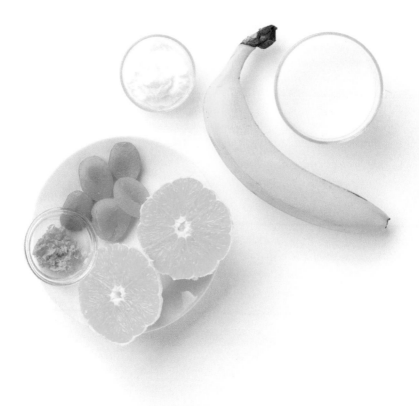

YOU NEED

1 banana, peeled and chopped • 1 orange, peeled • ⅔ cup rice milk
5 dried apricots • ¼ cup plain Greek yogurt
1 teaspoon finely grated orange zest

Dried apricots are full of dietary fiber, potassium, iron, and antioxidants.

D *Aids digestion* **B** *Bone strengthening* **E** *Energy boosting*

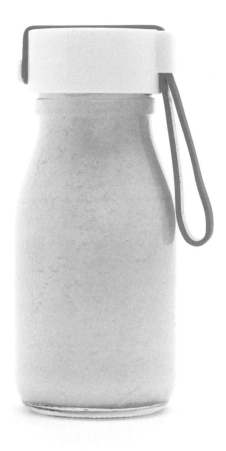

Place all the ingredients in a blender and blend until smooth.

INDEX

Entries in italics refer to recipe names.

A
açai powder 22, 32
Açai Seng 22
agave nectar 26
almond butter 78, 80, 102, 106, 110, 114, 116, 126, 144
Almond Joy 76
Almond Load 134
almond milk 14, 34, 36, 40, 48, 64, 76, 78, 80, 86, 90, 98, 104, 106, 114, 116, 132, 134, 140
almonds 40, 64, 76, 98, 134
apple juice 16, 38, 44
apples 74, 76, 84, 96, 102, 106, 150
apricots 156
arugula 136
avocado 34, 58, 82, 86, 90, 104, 138

B
Back in Black 138
banana 14, 16, 18, 20, 26, 28, 30, 40, 42, 52, 54, 56, 58, 60, 64, 66, 72, 76, 80, 82, 96, 104, 108, 110, 116, 118, 120, 122, 126, 128, 130, 132, 134, 136, 140, 146, 148, 152, 154, 156
Banana Nut 116
Banana Oat 40
basil 66
bee pollen 42, 86
beet 150
  juice 44
Beet Out 44
berries, mixed 32
Berry Scoop 32
black beans 138

Blue Apple 16
Blue Cashew 112
Blue Egg 34
blueberries 16, 34, 54, 56, 86, 112, 126, 136
bran flakes 136
Branberry Rocket 136
Brocco Bana 54
broccoli 54
Buckwheat Bang 154
buckwheat flakes 154

C
Cacao Delight 80
Cacao Flax 128
cacao nibs 20, 32, 80, 108, 118, 128, 146
cannellini beans 144
Caribbean Kick 104
carrots 44, 98, 150
cashew milk 20, 108, 112, 118
cashew nut butter 112
cashew nuts 64, 100
cherries 60
  juice 60
Cherry Bomb 60
Chia Charge 56
chia seeds 46, 56, 110, 118, 122
Chia Tea 46
Choc Espresso 20
cinnamon 48, 70, 102, 114, 130, 134, 142, 144
Coco Berry 24
Coco Melon 92
Coconut Date 14
coconut flakes 18
coconut meat 92
coconut milk 30, 102, 110, 120
coconut oil 28

coconut water 14, 16, 22, 24, 26, 46, 56, 64, 66, 82, 84, 136
coconut yogurt 24, 30, 94
coffee 20, 108
cranberries, dried 110
Cranberry Pro 110
cucumber 38

D
dates, Medjool, 14, 20, 28, 40, 48, 54, 58, 64, 78, 80, 86, 122, 128, 146, 154

E
eggs 34

F
Figgy Water 26
figs 26
flaxseed, ground 36, 52, 54, 58, 60, 64, 94, 128
flaxseed oil 34
Fruity Kale 96

G
ginger 44, 68, 74, 114
ginseng powder 22
goji berries 118
Grape Trifecta 62
grapes 62, 74, 84
  juice 62
Green Monster 84
Green Peach 68
Green Protein 106
green tea 46, 72, 74
Green Up 38

H
hazelnut milk 42
hazelnuts 64, 146
hemp seeds 58, 62, 104, 108, 110, 118

honey 22, 24, 68, 70, 74, 90, 92, 94, 100, 136, 138

J

jalapeño, pickled 104

K

kale 72, 96, 120, 150
Kale Kiwi Tea 72
kefir milk 74
kiwi 72, 100
Kiwi Raspberry 100

L

lemon juice 16, 46, 62, 150
lime juice 70, 104
Loca Mocha 108

M

maca powder 42, 118
Magic Mango 94
mango 18, 22, 42, 70, 86, 94, 104
Mango-Yo 70
Match Fit Maca 42
matcha (green tea) 36
melon 38, 92
milk kefir 74
mint 38

N

Nut Better 64
nutmeg 102
Nutty Boom 140

O

Oat & Tofu 90
Oat Me Up 146
oat milk 60, 96, 100, 146
oats 24, 40, 48, 66, 90, 94, 102, 112, 132, 134, 140, 146

Oaty Apple 102
Orangavo 58
Orange Tornado 142
oranges 58, 142, 156
Orangey Apricot 156

P

papaya 18, 28, 98, 148
Papaya Passion 98
Papaya Pine 18
passion fruit 98
Peach Carbler 126
Peachellini 144
peaches 32, 68, 126, 144
peanut butter 48, 64, 122
Peanut Chia 122
Peanut Spice 48
Pear Pro 36
pears 36, 96
pecans 140
Piña Coco Lada 28
Piña Spirulina 120
pineapple 22, 28, 32, 82, 120
pineapple juice 18
Pink Basil 66
Pollen Berry 86
Pom Flax-tastic 52
pomegranate juice 52
protein powder 32, 106, 112, 114, 116
Pumpkin Patch 114
pumpkin purée 114
pumpkin seeds 66, 114

R

raspberries 24, 78, 100
Raspberry Date 78
rice milk 52, 122, 130, 138, 142, 144, 150, 152, 154, 156

S

sea salt 64
soy milk 148
spinach 38, 52, 68, 84, 106, 126, 132, 134, 138
Spinachia 132
spirulina powder 86, 120
strawberries 30, 56, 66, 72, 96, 128
Super Goji 118
Sweet Papaya Poyo 148
Sweet Potana 152
sweet potato 130, 142, 148, 152
Sweet Potato Jive 130
Sweet-Kea 74

T

tofu, silken 90, 98
Tropical Turmeric 82
turmeric 82

V

vanilla extract 34, 48, 60, 116, 118
Veggie Beet 150

W

walnuts 140, 152
watermelon 94

Y

Yo Strawberries 30
yogurt 38, 58, 60, 66, 70, 78, 92, 96, 100, 114, 126, 128, 132, 136, 138, 140, 148, 154, 156

The author has researched each plant and superfood used in this book but is not responsible for any adverse effects any of the plants may have on an individual. One plant may be good for one person but have a negative effect on another. All the plants are consumed entirely at your own risk. Never use anything as an alternative to seeking professional medical advice and always consume in moderation. Nutrient analysis is based on USDA standard reference values or individual manufacturer's data.

Smoothies Du Sportif © Hachette Livre (Marabout), Paris, 2017
North American edition published by VeloPress, 2019

3002 Sterling Circle, Suite 100, Boulder, CO 80301 USA

VeloPress is the leading publisher of books on endurance sports and is a division of Pocket Outdoor Media. Focused on cycling, triathlon, running, swimming, and nutrition/diet, VeloPress books help athletes achieve their goals of going faster and farther. Preview books and contact us at velopress.com.

Distributed in the United States and Canada by Ingram Publisher Services

Library of Congress Cataloging-in-Publication Data
Names: Green, Fern, author.
Title: Sport smoothies : more than 65 recipes to boost your workouts & recovery / Fern Green ; photographs by Deirdre Rooney.
Other titles: Smoothies du sportif. English
Description: Boulder, Colorado : VeloPress, [2019] | Translation of: Smoothies du sportif. | Includes index. |
Identifiers: LCCN 2018049268 (print) | LCCN 2018049957 (ebook) | ISBN 9781948006156 (ebook) | ISBN 9781937715991 (pbk.)
Subjects: LCSH: Smoothies (Beverages) | Athletes–Nutrition. | LCGFT: Cookbooks.
Classification: LCC TX817.S636 (ebook) | LCC TX817.S636 G74613 2019 (print) | DDC 641.8/75–dc23
LC record available at https://lccn.loc.gov/2018049268

This paper meets the requirements of ANSI/NISO Z39.48-1992 (Permanence of Paper).

Photography by Deirdre Rooney
Design by Michelle Tilly

19 20 21 / 10 9 8 7 6 5 4 3 2 1